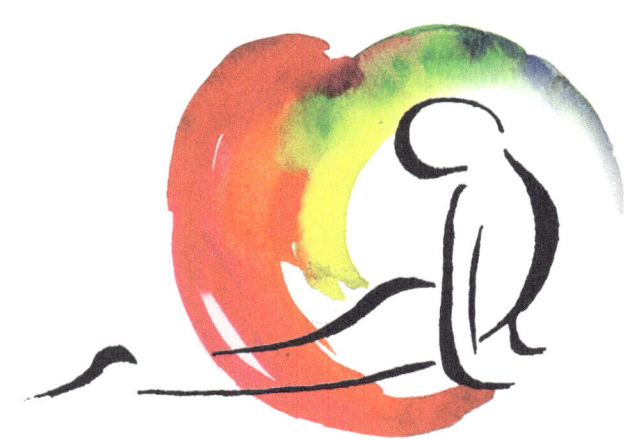

Yogagenda

PLANNER   HANDBOOK   JOURNAL

2014

www.YogagendaS.com

My personal info

_____

_____

_____

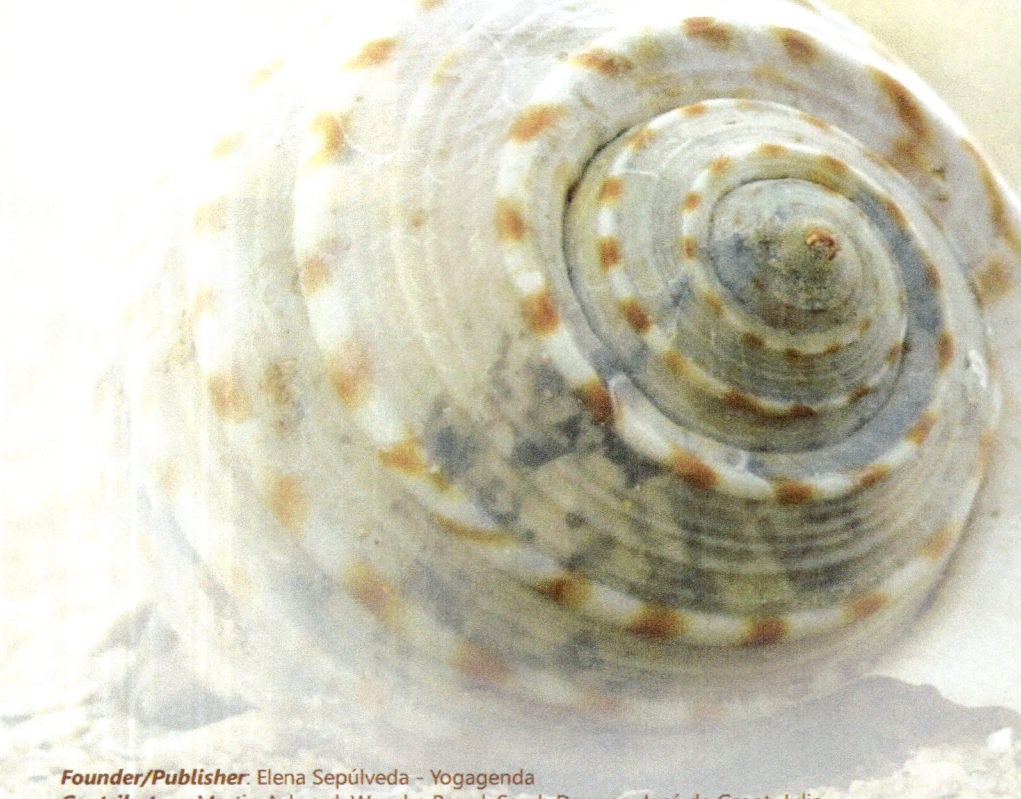

Founder/Publisher: Elena Sepúlveda - Yogagenda
Contributors: Martin Aylward, Wenche Beard, Sarah Dawson, José de Groot, Julie Hanson, Vidya Heisel, David Lurey, Mariah Mansvelt Beck, Irantzu Piquero, Swami Saradananda, Michelle Taffe, ShuKram Das, Mirjam Wagner, Sue Woodd
Graphic Design: José Macizo
Copy Editing: Gabrielle Green
Proofing: Claire Sutcliffe
Illustrators: Marta Giddings, Denise Ullmann
Front Cover: Image©Andrea Haase/Shutterstock.com

For more information or to place an order, please visit: www.YogagendaS.com

ISBN: 978-0-9572635-1-2

Disclaimer: The publisher, editor and all contributors disclaim any liability or loss in connection with the theories and practices offered in this *Yogagenda*.

Table Of Contents

What's In
YOGAGENDA 2014

Namaste and welcome to the third edition of *Yogagenda*! Whether you are a returning reader or this is your first time with us, I'm delighted to share with you this ever-evolving yoga publication. Putting together *Yogagenda* each year has become a yoga practice in itself: if the structure is akin to a specific sequence of asanas we repeat over a period of time, the contents are the changes we observe unfolding in ourselves within that sequence... Although this year's edition has a strong emphasis on "change", it does maintain untouched its fundamental structure with three distinct sections: the **YEARLY PLANNER**, the **YOGA HANDBOOK** and the **JOURNAL PAGES**.

I hope you enjoy what we are offering you this year. If you have any suggestions or would like to contribute to future editions of *Yogagenda*, please drop me an email or find me in any of the events I attend for *Yogagenda* in Europe.

And don't forget to visit **www.YogagendaS.com** for: more information about this project; an Inspiration section with book, DVD, film and music suggestions; links to our teacher and healer friends; and a great on-line shop to purchase copies of all *Yogagenda*'s editions.

May 2014 brings you endless blessings.

Elena Sepúlveda
Yogagenda Editor
elena@YogagendaS.com

YEARLY PLANNER

We are all about being practical.

This section includes:

- **2 Year-at-a-Glance Calendars** (one for 2014 and another for 2015)
- **1 "Closing the Year 2013/ Welcoming the Year 2014" double spread**. You may find this useful to reflect on the direction your life is taking, or to recap and plan ahead as one year comes to an end and the next one begins.
- **12 Mohth-at-a-Glance Calendars**, one per page, with space for notes.
- **52 Week-at-a-Glance Calendars**, with a week on two pages. Weeks are numbered from one to 52, and each weekly double spread contains a small month-at-a-glance calendar, plus information on **moon phases, solstices, equinoxes** and **solar/lunar eclipses** for 2014. As we are based in Europe, we have followed a Northern Hemisphere perspective; if you read us from a different part of the planet, please visit **www.timeanddate.com** for information more relevant to you.

YOGA HANDBOOK

We are all about being informative and, hopefully, inspirational.

At the core of the 2014 contributions there is a focus on change, on the cycle of the seasons and on striking a balance between theory and practice. All *Yogagenda* contributors are experts in their fields. Coming from at least 10 different countries and working all over the world from Barcelona to Byron Bay, Amsterdam to Israel or the Caribbean to Crete, they are practising yoga teachers living and breathing within the yogic community worldwide. To find out more about them and their work, please go to **Who Contributed to Yogagenda 2014** (pp.238-241).

This section includes:

- **12 Monthly Symbols**, illustrated by Marta Moia and written by Elena Sepúlveda. This year's symbolism is inspired by the Five Daoist Elements underlying the practice of Yin yoga: Water, Wood, Fire, Earth and Metal. In this model of the cyclical nature of the universe, Water (rain/winter) makes Wood (plants/spring) grow which in turn are scorched by Fire (heat/summer) to then turn to Earth (ashes/late summer); within the Earth, Metal (cold/autumn) ores are formed which, when cold, causes Water to condense, bringing about the rain that will start the creative cycle anew. As you move through the different months of the year, we'd like to offer you a small reflection token to help attune with the energy of each season. May nature and change be our teachers!

- **Asana Overview: Yin Asanas for All Seasons**, by Elena Sepúlveda. This spread describes the criteria followed for grouping this year's yoga poses: the five seasons of Chinese medicine which are at the core of Yin yoga, and how these relate to the meridians or "energy paths" in our body and their associated internal organs. Most of these asanas come together in **The Sequence: Yin for the Spine** (see below).
- **Asana Pages**, illustrated by Denise Ullmann and written by Elena Sepúlveda. There is one colour and symbol-coded Yin asana per month, with concise instructions on how to get into and exit the pose, a suggested holding time, the meridians and organs it affects, its anatomical benefits and contra-indications, some variations and a Yang yoga version of each pose.

- **Seasonal Energy: Balancing Change**. Sue Woodd and Julie Hanson offer very practical suggestions to help you tune into each month's and season's energy.
- **The Body of Life: Inhabiting Our Practice**. Martin Aylward on the transformative power of yoga that comes from inhabiting our body and practice.
- **Meditation: A Practical Perspective**. Swami Saradananda on how to make a daily meditation practice a reality.
- **Yoga beyond the Mat: The Choclo Project**. Elena Sepúlveda on a beautiful project that brings together underprivileged children in Peru and yoga clothing in a highly creative and ethical way.
- **Yin & Yang Yoga: the Perfect Combo**. José de Groot on the main differences between these two kinds of yoga and how they coexist in a balanced practice.
- **The Koshas: Unleashing Yoga's Potential**. Sarah Dawson on how to enhance your yoga practice by being mindful of our body's koshas.
- **Mantra and Vibration: A Divine Path to Union**. David Lurey on the liberating effect of chanting and Bhakti yoga.

- **Durga: The Goddess of a Thousand Faces**. Irantzu Piquero on the disappearance of the Goddess figure and her subsequent return in her most fierce aspect.
- **Fascia: The Glue that Holds our Body Together**. Mirjam Wagner on this often neglected tissue that wraps every single one of our muscles and nerve fibres.
- **Yoga in the First Person: Dancing to Kali's Energy**. Wenche Beard's personal account of how embracing her shadows through her yoga practice led her to fully fall in love with life.
- **To Eat or not to Eat: A Yogic Diet**. Vidya Heisel on how yogic traditional dietary advice relates (or not) to our present-day lives.
- **Hanuman: The Breath within the Breath**. ShuKram Das on the yoga teachings behind the Monkey-God story in the Indian epic Ramayana.
- **The Sequence: Yin for the Spine**. Devised by Mariah Mansvelt Beck and illustrated by Denise Ullman, this Yin yoga sequence focuses on stretching and stimulating the entire spine in a slow and mindful manner.
- **Yoga Festivals & Celebrations around the Globe**. Michelle Taffe of The Global Yogi once again brings us her well-researched listing of yoga events around the world in 2014.
- **Sanskrit Glossary**. These pages offer short explanations of the Sanskrit terms used in this edition of *Yogagenda*.
- **Asana Index**. This page provides you with a quick way to find the Yin and Yang poses included in the Asana Pages.
- **Patanjali's Yoga Sutras**. Each week includes a sutra in Sanskrit from the third chapter of Patanjali's Yoga Sutras. Translations into English for these and the first and second chapters (published in 2012 and 2013 respectively) can be found at **www.YogagendaS.com**.

JOURNAL PAGES

We are all about encouraging creative reflection.

This section includes:
- Journal or blank pages integrated at different points in the agenda (and more at the end too). They are blank sheets for your own needs: to do some planning, to spread your creative wings on paper, to reflect on the topics introduced in the articles, or for whatever takes your fancy.

Closing the year 2013

Welcoming the year 2014

2014

January

	1	2	3	4	**5**
6	7	8	9	10	11	**12**
13	14	15	16	17	18	**19**
20	21	22	23	24	25	**26**
27	28	29	30	31		

February

					1	**2**
3	4	5	6	7	8	**9**
10	11	12	13	14	15	**16**
17	18	19	20	21	22	**23**
24	25	26	27	28		

March

					1	**2**
3	4	5	6	7	8	**9**
10	11	12	13	14	15	**16**
17	18	19	20	21	22	**23**
24	25	26	27	28	29	**30**
31						

April

	1	2	3	4	5	**6**
7	8	9	10	11	12	**13**
14	15	16	17	18	19	**20**
21	22	23	24	25	26	**27**
28	29	30				

May

			1	2	3	**4**
5	6	7	8	9	10	**11**
12	13	14	15	16	17	**18**
19	20	21	22	23	24	**25**
26	27	28	29	30	31	

June

						1
2	3	4	5	6	7	**8**
9	10	11	12	13	14	**15**
16	17	18	19	20	21	**22**
23	24	25	26	27	28	**29**
30						

July

	1	2	3	4	5	**6**
7	8	9	10	11	12	**13**
14	15	16	17	18	19	**20**
21	22	23	24	25	26	**27**
28	29	30	31			

August

				1	2	**3**
4	5	6	7	8	9	**10**
11	12	13	14	15	16	**17**
18	19	20	21	22	23	**24**
25	26	27	28	29	30	**31**

September

1	2	3	4	5	6	**7**
8	9	10	11	12	13	**14**
15	16	17	18	19	20	**21**
22	23	24	25	26	27	**28**
29	30					

October

	1	2	3	4		**5**
6	7	8	9	10	11	**12**
13	14	15	16	17	18	**19**
20	21	22	23	24	25	**26**
27	28	29	30	31		

November

					1	**2**
3	4	5	6	7	8	**9**
10	11	12	13	14	15	**16**
17	18	19	20	21	22	**23**
24	25	26	27	28	29	**30**

December

1	2	3	4	5	6	**7**
8	9	10	11	12	13	**14**
15	16	17	18	19	20	**21**
22	23	24	25	26	27	**28**
29	30	31				

2015

January
		1	2	3	**4**
5	6	7	8	9	10	**11**
12	13	14	15	16	17	**18**
19	20	21	22	23	24	**25**
26	27	28	29	30	31

February
						1
2	3	4	5	6	7	**8**
9	10	11	12	13	14	**15**
16	17	18	19	20	21	**22**
23	24	25	26	27	28

March
						1
2	3	4	5	6	7	**8**
9	10	11	12	13	14	**15**
16	17	18	19	20	21	**22**
23	24	25	26	27	28	**29**
30	31

April
		1	2	3	4	**5**
6	7	8	9	10	11	**12**
13	14	15	16	17	18	**19**
20	21	22	23	24	25	**26**
27	28	29	30

May
				1	2	**3**
4	5	6	7	8	9	**10**
11	12	13	14	15	16	**17**
18	19	20	21	22	23	**24**
25	26	27	28	29	30	**31**

June
1	2	3	4	5	6	**7**
8	9	10	11	12	13	**14**
15	16	17	18	19	20	**21**
22	23	24	25	26	27	**28**
29	30

July
	1	2	3	4	**5**
6	7	8	9	10	11	**12**
13	14	15	16	17	18	**19**
20	21	22	23	24	25	**26**
27	28	29	30	31

August
					1	**2**
3	4	5	6	7	8	**9**
10	11	12	13	14	15	**16**
17	18	19	20	21	22	**23**
24	25	26	27	28	29	**30**
31

September
	1	2	3	4	5	**6**
7	8	9	10	11	12	**13**
14	15	16	17	18	19	**20**
21	22	23	24	25	26	**27**
28	29	30

October
		1	2	3	**4**
5	6	7	8	9	10	**11**
12	13	14	15	16	17	**18**
19	20	21	22	23	24	**25**
26	27	28	29	30	31

November
						1
2	3	4	5	6	7	**8**
9	10	11	12	13	14	**15**
16	17	18	19	20	21	**22**
23	24	25	26	27	28	**29**
30

December
	1	2	3	4	5	**6**
7	8	9	10	11	12	**13**
14	15	16	17	18	19	**20**
21	22	23	24	25	26	**27**
28	29	30	31

January 2014

Monday	Tuesday	Wednesday	Thursday	Friday	Saturday	Sunday
		○ 1	2	3	4	5
6	7	☽ 8	9	10	11	12
13	14	15	○ 16 Micro Moon	17	18	19
20	21	22	23	☾ 24	25	26
27	28	29	○ 30	31		

February 2014

Monday	Tuesday	Wednesday	Thursday	Friday	Saturday	Sunday
					1	2
3	4	5	☽ 6	7	8	9
10	11	12	13	○ 14	15	16
17	18	19	20	21	☽ 22	23
24	25	26	27	28		

March 2014

Monday	Tuesday	Wednesday	Thursday	Friday	Saturday	Sunday
					○ 1	2
3	4	5	6	7	☽ 8	9
10	11	12	13	14	15	○ 16
17	18	19	20 Spring Equinox	21	22	23
☾ 24	25	26	27	28	29	○ 30
31						

April 2014

Monday	Tuesday	Wednesday	Thursday	Friday	Saturday	Sunday
	1	2	3	4	5	6
☽ 7	8	9	10	11	12	13
14	○ 15 Total Lunar Eclipse	16	17	18	19	20
21	☾ 22	23	24	25	26	27
28	○ 29 Annular Solar Eclipse	30				

May 2014

Monday	Tuesday	Wednesday	Thursday	Friday	Saturday	Sunday
			1	2	3	4
5	6	☽ 7	8	9	10	11
12	13	○ 14	15	16	17	18
19	20	☾ 21	22	23	24	25
26	27	○ 28	29	30	31	

June 2014

Monday	Tuesday	Wednesday	Thursday	Friday	Saturday	Sunday
						1
2	3	4	☽ 5	6	7	8
9	10	11	12	○ 13	14	15
16	17	18	☾ 19	20	21 Summer Solstice	22
23	24	25	26	○ 27	28	29
30						

July 2014

Monday	Tuesday	Wednesday	Thursday	Friday	Saturday	Sunday
	1	2	3	4	☽ 5	6
7	8	9	10	11	○ 12	13
14	15	16	17	18	☾ 19	20
21	22	23	24	25	○ 26	27
28	29	30	31			

August 2014

Monday	Tuesday	Wednesday	Thursday	Friday	Saturday	Sunday
				1	2	3
☽ 4	5	6	7	8	9	○ 10 Super Full Moon
11	12	13	14	15	16	☾ 17
18	19	20	21	22	23	24
○ 25	26	27	28	29	30	31

September 2014

Monday	Tuesday	Wednesday	Thursday	Friday	Saturday	Sunday
1	☽ 2	3	4	5	6	7
8	○ 9	10	11	12	13	14
15	☾ 16	17	18	19	20	21
22	23 Autumn Equinox	○ 24	25	26	27	28
29	30					

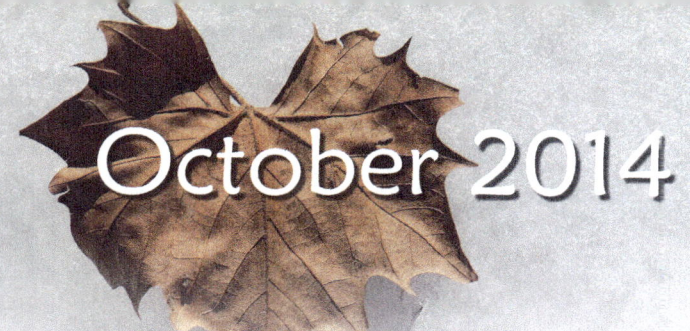

October 2014

Monday	Tuesday	Wednesday	Thursday	Friday	Saturday	Sunday
		☽ 1	2	3	4	5
6	7	◯ 8 Total Lunar Eclipse	9	10	11	12
13	14	☾ 15	16	17	18	19
20	21	22	◯ 23 Partial Solar Eclipse	24	25	26
27	28	29	30	☽ 31		

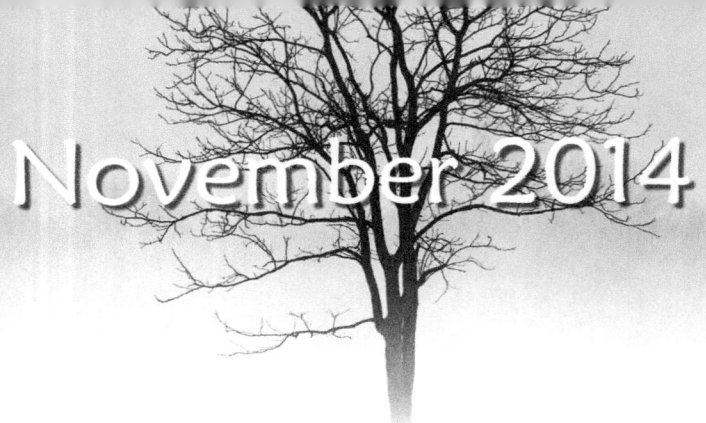

November 2014

Monday	Tuesday	Wednesday	Thursday	Friday	Saturday	Sunday
					1	2
3	4	5	○ 6	7	8	9
10	11	12	13	☾ 14	15	16
17	18	19	20	21	○ 22	23
24	25	26	27	28	☽ 29	30

December 2014

Monday	Tuesday	Wednesday	Thursday	Friday	Saturday	Sunday
1	2	3	4	5	○ 6	7
8	9	10	11	12	13	☾ 14
15	16	17	18	19	20	21
○ 22 Winter Solstice	23	24	25	26	27	☽ 28
29	30	31				

Asana Overview:
YIN ASANAS FOR ALL SEASONS

By Elena Sepúlveda

You are probably reading this in winter. Unlike the leafless trees in your neighbourhood, you are clad in quite a few layers of clothing and your energy (just like the trees') is drawn inwards as a result of days being short and light scarce. It's time to slow down, to be quieter, to recharge our batteries. Our yoga practice is different from our practice on a hot summer's day because our energy levels are not the same. The benefits from being attuned to the changes in nature (including our own nature!) are huge. With this in mind, our asanas for this year's edition of *Yogagenda* have a seasonal (see article on Seasonal Energy; pp.40-43) as well as a Yin yoga (see article on Yin & Yang Yoga; pp.106-109) perspective.

Yin yoga is based on Chinese medicine, where the cycle of life has five seasons associated with five elements: Winter - Water, Spring - Wood, Summer - Fire, Late Summer - Earth, and Autumn - Metal. Each season's element is also associated with two internal organs with complementary functions: a yin or hollow organ and a yang or solid organ. And those internal organs are connected by a network of meridians or "electromagnetic paths" that conduct energy throughout the body; organs and meridians are inseparable. Our internal organs have a physical function, but also an energetic and a psychological one. If our organs are weak and we lack vital energy, our emotions will suffer. And vice versa: if our emotions are out of balance, we can become tired and physically ill. By making energy flow through the meridians so our organs improve function, we become healthy physically as well as emotionally.

Both internal organs and meridians can be affected by specific Yin yoga asanas. This gentle practice with long-held poses stimulates the vital energy or chi that flows throughout the fascia (see article on Fascia; pp.172-175), where the meridians are situated, contributing to overall health and wellbeing. Long-held Yin yoga poses also allow us to fully inhabit our body (see article on The Body of Life; pp.56-59), and accept it independently of whether we are feeling pain or pleasure. Remaining for a few minutes in an asana gives us a chance to investigate any possible emotional blockages, and to become wiser. When you exit the pose as gently and mindfully as you entered it, you generate a truly meditative state (see article on Meditation; pp.72-75) and further opportunity for observation and union (yoga).

You'll find most of the following featured poses coming together in The Sequence: Yin for the Spine (pp.228-231).

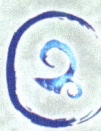

Winter Poses

Internal organs: kidneys (yang) and urinary bladder (yin).
Asanas for the Kidney meridian: **Squat** (pp.222-223) and **Saddle** (pp.38-39).
Asana for the Urinary Bladder meridian: **Snail** (pp.54-55).

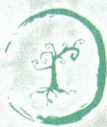

Spring Poses

Internal organs: liver (yang) and gall bladder (yin).
Asanas for the Liver meridian: **Stirrup** (pp.70-71) and **Square** (pp.88-89).
Asana for the Gall Bladder meridian: **Butterfly** (pp.104-105).

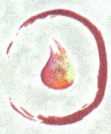

Summer Poses

Internal organs: heart (yang) and small intestine (yin).
Asana for the Heart meridian: **Anahatasana** (pp.120-121).
Asana for the Small Intestine meridian: **Reclining Twist** (pp.138-139).

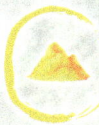

Late Summer Poses

Internal organs: spleen (yang) and stomach (yin).
Asana for the Spleen meridian: **Sphinx** (pp.154-155).
Asana for the Stomach meridian: **Dragon Flying High** (pp.170-171).

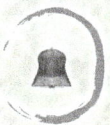

Autumn Poses

Internal organs: lungs (yang) and large intestine (yin).
Asana for the Lung meridian: **Bananasana with Arms Up** (pp.188-189).
Asana for the Large Intestine meridian: **Dragonfly Twist** (pp.204-205).

When describing the poses, we have emphasised their physical and energetic effects. However, like all yoga poses, they also have inherent emotional, mental and spiritual dimensions worth exploring more in depth.

Please bear in mind that not all poses and variations are suitable for all people. It is your responsibility to know your body and its limitations, and to choose a practice that is appropriate for you.

MOON – Water

The Moon influences the Earth's underground currents and rules over all flowing waters, from the tides of the ocean to our bodily fluids and those of plants and animals. As opposed to the Sun, which is associated with the masculine or yang, light and activity, the Moon is linked to the feminine or yin, darkness and passivity in many cultures – though not all. The Moon produces no light of itself; however, it reflects the Sun's light to bring clarity to the night. Attuning our energies to those of the Moon's phases may also bring clarity to us in the form of subtle understanding or intuition. These energies are: waning moon – time of incubation, contemplation, surrender; new moon – time for new beginnings, rebirth and fresh starts; waxing moon – time for growth and manifestation; full moon – the peak of clarity, fullness and the attainment of our desires.

January 2014

January 2014

		1	2	3	4	5
6	7	8	9	10	11	12
13	14	15	16	17	18	19
20	21	22	23	24	25	26
27	28	29	30	31		

30
MONDAY

31
TUESDAY

1
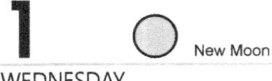 New Moon

WEDNESDAY

Patanjali's Yoga Sutras – Chapter III: Vibhuti Pada

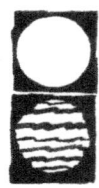

2
THURSDAY

3
FRIDAY

4
SATURDAY

5
SUNDAY

January 2014

						week 1
	1	2	3	4	5	week 1
6	7	8	9	10	11	12
13	14	15	16	17	18	19
20	21	22	23	24	25	26
27	28	29	30	31		

January 2014

6
MONDAY

7
TUESDAY

8
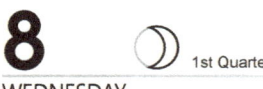 1st Quarter
WEDNESDAY

Sutra III.1 *desabandhas cittasya dharana*

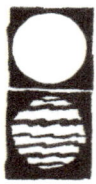

9
THURSDAY

10
FRIDAY

11
SATURDAY

12
SUNDAY

January 2014

	1	2	3	4	5
6	7	8	9	10	11	12
13	14	15	16	17	18	19
20	21	22	23	24	25	26
27	28	29	30	31		

week 2

January 2014

13
MONDAY

14
TUESDAY

15
WEDNESDAY

Sutra III.2 *tatra pratyayaikatanata dhyanam*

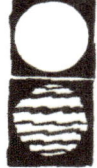

January 2014

Full Moon ○ **16**
Micro Moon **THURSDAY**

17
FRIDAY

18
SATURDAY

19
SUNDAY

January 2014

		1	2	3	4	5
6	7	8	9	10	11	12
13	14	15	16	17	18	19
20	21	22	23	24	25	26
27	28	29	30	31		

week 3

20
MONDAY

21
TUESDAY

22
WEDNESDAY

Sutra III.3 *tad evarthamatra nirbhasam svarupa sunyam iva samadhih*

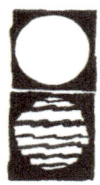

23
THURSDAY

Last Quarter  **24**
FRIDAY

25
SATURDAY

26
SUNDAY

January 2014

		1	2	3	4	5
6	7	8	9	10	11	12
13	14	15	16	17	18	19
20	21	22	23	24	25	26
27	28	29	30	31		

week 4

January 2014

27
MONDAY

28
TUESDAY

29
WEDNESDAY

Sutra III.4 *trayam ekatra samyamah*

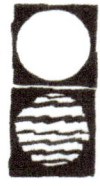

New Moon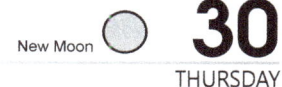

30
THURSDAY

31
FRIDAY

1
SATURDAY

2
SUNDAY

January 2014

		1	2	3	4	5
6	7	8	9	10	11	12
13	14	15	16	17	18	19
20	21	22	23	24	25	26
27	28	29	30	31		

week 5

SADDLE
Kidney Meridian

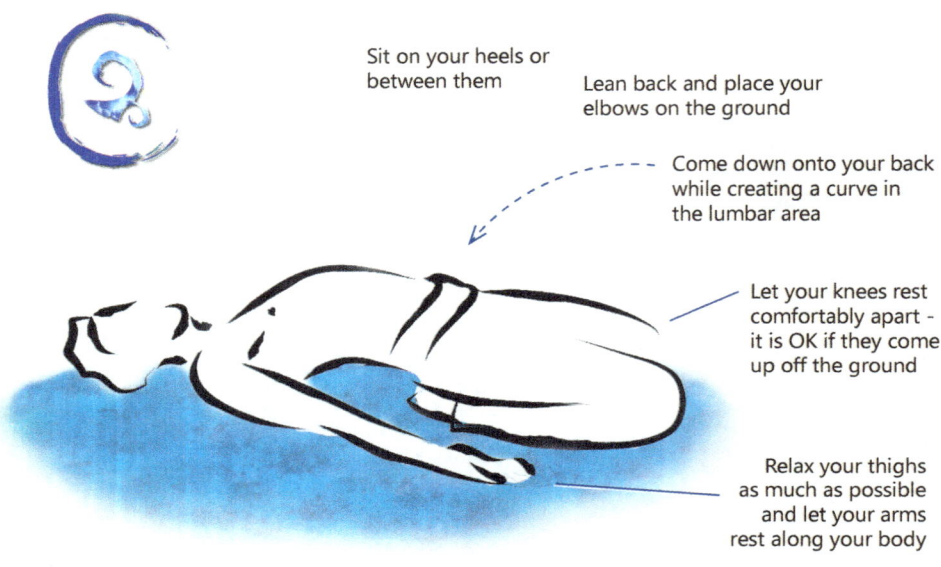

Sit on your heels or between them

Lean back and place your elbows on the ground

Come down onto your back while creating a curve in the lumbar area

Let your knees rest comfortably apart - it is OK if they come up off the ground

Relax your thighs as much as possible and let your arms rest along your body

While in the Pose

- Holding time: 1 to 5 minutes.
- Breathe deeply and mindfully.

Coming out of the Pose

- Leave the pose slowly and mindfully.
- Place your hands on the ground next to your body. Inhale, engage your abdominal muscles to protect your lumbar area and come back up to a sitting position. Lie on your belly with your legs relaxed and stretched out.
- Observe the effects of the pose.

Modifications and Variations

- If too much tension is felt in the sacral area or the ground is difficult to reach, place a cushion under your shoulders leaving your lower back unsupported.
- If you have lower back injuries, place a bolster or blanket length-wise supporting the whole back.
- Alternatively, don't go all the way and lean on your hands, forearms or elbows.

Taking it Further

- Stretch your arms overhead to open up your chest and shoulders.
- Sit between your ankles and extend one leg once your back is on the ground.

Meridians and Organs Affected

The Kidney, Stomach and Spleen meridians (front of torso and inner and front of legs).
The Urinary Bladder meridian (lumbar spine).
It stimulates the kidneys themselves and the thyroid gland if the neck drops back.

Anatomical Benefits

It stretches the abdomen, chest and hips.
It deeply stretches the thighs and the ankles.
It creates healthy stress in the lumbar area and allows you to move the sacrum.

Contraindications

Acute pain in the ankles or knees.
Not recommended when the sacrum is tight or has any injuries.

Yang Sibling

Supta Virasana (Reclining Hero Pose) or Supta Vajrasana (Reclining Thunderbolt Pose). In the Yang yoga versions of this pose, we tuck the tailbone in to keep the sacral area as close to the floor as possible.

If you feel any painful sensation in your sacrum, knees, ankles, or feet, use a variation of the pose!

MY NOTES

Seasonal Energy: BALANCING CHANGE

By Sue Woodd and Julie Hanson

We are a part of nature and therefore part of its changes, although it is probably easier for us to be aware of these changes in our animals or gardens than in ourselves. The changes brought about by each season are the essence of personal development and healing.

As we open our minds and look at how the world works, we can see that the body has homeostatic mechanisms for internal balancing, just as nature does. With too much internal (personal) and external (social) tension we can damage and create imbalances in our systems, thus draining our vital energy and working against natural energy flows.

Most of us don't necessarily know how to properly re-establish balance, and how to work with the seasonal cycles to put energy back into our systems. Rather than getting caught up in complicated scientific solutions, the solution can be simple changes in exercise, diet and lifestyle that can have the most profound effects on our health, self-esteem and well-being.

Here are some suggestions to help you tune into each month and each individual season's energy.

January
IMAGINATION AND DIRECTION

- Go to bed earlier and get up later (if possible). It's a time for rest and renewal!
- Do not go on a diet at this time of year, just simply clean up your act!
- Pay attention and listen to what people (and your inner guidance) are telling you.
- Find new determination to face your fears and make a plan to try to overcome them, but don't take any action yet.

February
VISIONS AND DECISIONS

- Take up meditation at least once a day for 10 minutes. Space and a still mind are the greatest catalysts for change and creativity.
- Treat yourself to as many massages as possible, to detox and promote the circulation to your muscles.
- Do you have a picture of how you would like to live and does the reality correspond to the picture? Find a quiet place where you can relax undisturbed and paint in details of how you would like to live your life, without restrictions and limitations, and keep adding to it!

March
GROWTH AND EXPANSION

- Spring clean half the house (up-stairs?), and the other half in April.
- Start walking outside in the new oxygenated air.
- Be kind to someone every day.
- Set three new goals, things that will enhance your life this year, and think of two things you can do to move you in the direction of each of your desired goals, and do them immediately!

April
JOY, PLEASURE AND PROTECTION

- Do the other half of the spring-cleaning (the downstairs).
- Practise speaking from the heart: being cordial, affectionate, enthusiastic and humorous.
- Make sure you are putting into action plans made in January!
- Try on last year's summer wardrobe and give away anything you haven't worn in the last year.

May
SUPPLENESS, STRENGTH AND CONNECTION

- Become more flexible in life; rigid in body is rigid in mind.
- Remember: you are what you eat, digest, absorb and eliminate mentally, emotionally and physically!
- Work on the health of the three levels of mind, emotions and body.
- Communicate your needs and ideas.

June
EXPRESSION AND ABSORPTION

- Take up brisk walking or running outside.
- Temper your desire to say "yes" with occasional "nos".
- Keep life simple and cultivate discernment this month! Is it necessary?
- Are you clear about what is important in your life? Make sure you don't just take on the convictions and beliefs of others undigested.

July
FIRE, EXPRESSION AND INSPIRATION

- Have a party, be more sociable and allow for self-expression.
- Cultivate the ability to give and receive warmth.
- List the things that open your heart, inspire you and develop appreciation.
- Have an afternoon nap then stay up a little later to make up for the lost time during the afternoon.

August
THOUGHTS AND NOURISHMENT

- Become aware of your personal concerns: what you reflect upon, agonise over and dream about.
- Make life more simple and harmonious.
- Work on relationships.
- Guard the quality of your thoughts. Are they supporting you?

September
BACK TO YOURSELF

- How much time do you have for yourself and your personal interests? Make sure you have enough; if not, schedule it in!
- Rub lotion into the body upward towards the heart to stimulate the lymphatic system and to get the immune system to optimum level before the autumn.
- Good time for studying, digesting information and life.
- Try to build a high sense of self-esteem at this point of the year.

October
STRUCTURE, STRENGTH AND DISCIPLINE

- Buy a dry skin body brush, use every morning before your shower.
- If something or someone is bugging you, now is the time to tell them, deal with it and get it off your chest.
- Hold on to your principles and keep your commitments.
- Look out for depression, it can often happen at this time of year; breathe well, don't collapse your chest and hold your head up high.

November
JUDGEMENT, CLARITY AND OPENNESS

- Burn lots of spicy aromatherapy oils in the house; it's the time when the sense of smell is at a peak.
- Clear up misunderstandings and focus on what's important and what you value.
- At home, clear out clutter.
- Get your finances in order.

December
REFLECTIVE, PROFOUND AND COURAGEOUS

- Use your imagination and give yourself time to think and reflect.
- Who do you respect and revere?
- Avoid the tendency to overdo things and become totally exhausted!
- Keep your kidneys warm, wrap up around your back area.

MY NOTES

SHELL – Water

Found in oceans, on river beds and beaches, shells are a traditional symbol of water and (re)birth. Aphrodite, the Greek goddess of love and beauty, is born from the ocean's waters riding on a shell. One of the eight auspicious symbols of Buddhism is a conch shell; it represents the sound of the Dharma (or Buddhist teachings) reaching far and wide, liberating beings from the muddy waters of greed, hatred and ignorance. A conch shell is also used as a trumpet to convert breath into life-giving sound in Hinduism, where Vishnu, as Lord of the Waters, issued from one the primordial creative sound: OM. Keeping a shell at home can remind us to practise conscious breathing; we also came to this life with an in-breath – and will leave it with an out-breath! As meditation teacher Thich Nhat Hanh says, "breath is the bridge that connects life to consciousness."

February 2014

JOURNAL

February 2014

					1	2
3	4	5	6	7	8	9
10	11	12	13	14	15	16
17	18	19	20	21	22	23
24	25	26	27	28		

PLANNER HANDBOOK JOURNAL | 45

February 2014

3
MONDAY

4
TUESDAY

5
WEDNESDAY

Sutra III.5 *tajjayat prajnalokah*

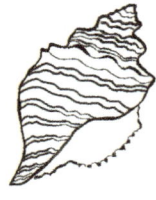

February 2014

First Quarter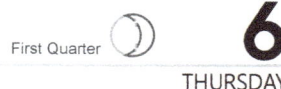

6
THURSDAY

7
FRIDAY

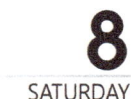
8
SATURDAY

9
SUNDAY

February 2014

					1	2
3	4	5	6	7	8	9	week 6
10	11	12	13	14	15	16
17	18	19	20	21	22	23
24	25	26	27	28		

February 2014

10
MONDAY

11
TUESDAY

12
WEDNESDAY

Sutra III.6 *tasya bhumisu viniyogah*

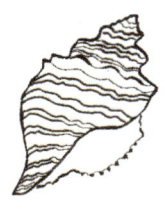

13
THURSDAY

Full Moon ◯ **14**
FRIDAY

15
SATURDAY

16
SUNDAY

February 2014

					1	2
3	4	5	6	7	8	9
10	11	12	13	14	15	16
17	18	19	20	21	22	23
24	25	26	27	28		

week 7

February 2014

17
MONDAY

18
TUESDAY

19
WEDNESDAY

Sutra III.7 *trayam antarangam purvebhyah*

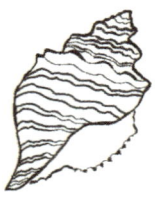

February 2014

20
THURSDAY

21
FRIDAY

Last Quarter 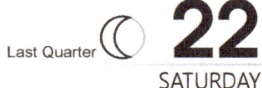 ## 22
SATURDAY

23
SUNDAY

February 2014

						1	2
3	4	5	6	7	8	9	
10	11	12	13	14	15	16	
17	18	19	20	21	22	23	
24	25	26	27	28			

week 8

February 2014

24
MONDAY

25
TUESDAY

26
WEDNESDAY

Sutra III.8 *tad api bahirangam mirbijasya*

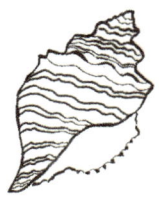

27

THURSDAY

28

FRIDAY

New Moon 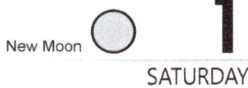 **1**

SATURDAY

2

SUNDAY

February 2014

					1	2
3	4	5	6	7	8	9
10	11	12	13	14	15	16
17	18	19	20	21	22	23
24	25	26	27	28		

week 9

SNAIL
Urinary Bladder Meridian

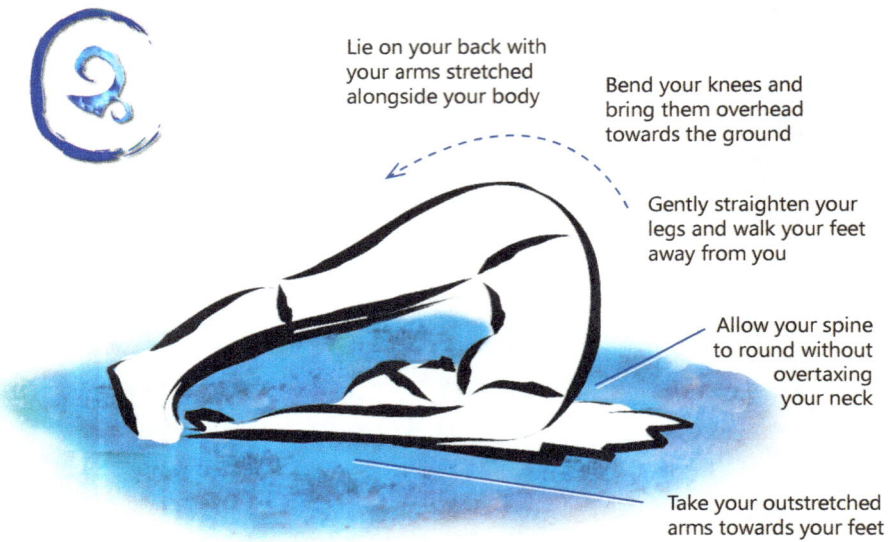

Lie on your back with your arms stretched alongside your body

Bend your knees and bring them overhead towards the ground

Gently straighten your legs and walk your feet away from you

Allow your spine to round without overtaxing your neck

Take your outstretched arms towards your feet

While in the Pose

- Holding time: 3 to 5 minutes.
- Breathe deeply and mindfully.

Coming out of the Pose

- Leave the pose slowly and mindfully.
- Place your hands on the ground alongside your body. As you exhale, roll your back to the ground using your abdominal muscles to control the descent.
- Lie on your back with your knees bent and feet flat on the ground while moving your head gently from side to side.
- Observe the effects of the pose.

Modifications and Variations

- Keep your hands on your back if your feet don't reach the ground.
- To lessen the pressure on the neck, place neatly folded blankets at the edge of your shoulders so that the neck vertebrae are less compressed.

Taking it Further

- Take your arms back to their initial position alongside your body and clasp your hands together.
- Drop your knees towards the ground to either side of your ears, rounding the spine more deeply.
- Place your hands on your legs and slowly start to roll out of the pose while using the weight of your arms as breaks.

Meridians and Organs Affected

The Urinary Bladder meridian (lumbar and dorsal spine).
It massages the stomach, heart and all other internal organs.

Anatomical Benefits

It deeply releases the muscles and ligaments along the whole spine.

Contraindications

Neck problems.
This pose is an inversion and should be avoided if your blood pressure is very high.
Not recommended during pregnancy.

Yang Sibling

Halasana (Plough Pose). In the Yang yoga version of this pose, the legs are active and we try to keep the spine long rather than rounded, and the hips high.

If you feel any painful sensation in your neck, use a variation of the pose!

MY NOTES

The Body Of Life:
INHABITING OUR PRACTICE

By Martin Aylward

Are you able to notice "the basic aliveness of bodily life"? The essence of yoga is the internalisation of your attention; to be inside of every posture, to inhabit every breath, emotion or movement... That is the truly transformative power of yoga.

There is a line in James Joyce's *Dubliners*, which describes to the reader how "Mr Duffy lived a short distance from his body". We all know the experience of being entangled in our inner stories and abstractions, divorced from our immediate, lived experience. It is just this separation from our selves, this gap between where our life is and where our attention is, that yoga ultimately exists to dissolve. As London Underground reminds its passengers: "Mind the Gap". The "Union" that is the root meaning of the word "yoga", is this re-union, this resolution of what we call my life, and life itself, of heart, mind and body, of self and world.

How is your body feeling as you read this? How close is your attention to your direct, felt experience? Is it, like poor Mr Duffy, some-where out ahead of you, entranced by the activity of your mind, at the expense of bodily immediacy? We tend to read with our minds, and we may not be able to even imagine another way of doing it. There is something crucial however about staying in touch with our visceral experience, moment by moment. Whatever yoga tradition we may practise in, the fundamental ground of yoga, prior to posture and breath, and certainly more primary than how far we stretch or how toned we are, is this direct contact with bodily life. To really inhabit your posture is to train your attention to be right where you are, to listen deeply to your life, to open the antenna of awareness to the intimate and unerring signals that are playing out in the dance of sensation and vibration that we call bodily life.

We tend to think we already know what this body is. This assumed knowledge, whether of body or anything else in life, fundamentally limits us from actually finding out, in the intimacy and immediacy of our current experience, what is actually happening. Common sense tells me about my body in terms of its shape, size and gender, supported by what I can see of it, and the mental image I have of it. But let us look for the rather uncommon sense of direct perception, to put aside what we think we know in order to really find out: what is this that I call body?

As you read these words, let yourself just sense your body sitting here; the weight of your legs and buttocks on the chair or cushion, the felt sense of your posture as you sense it from the inside. Notice if there are any subtle tension patterns revealed in this bodily awareness and in noticing them, see if they can yield to the intention to let them soften and relax.

Above all, notice the basic aliveness of bodily life. Allow the fluidity of sensation, the naturalness of the rhythm and movement of breathing. Let this fundamental aliveness be the centre of your experience. More than our changing thoughts, more than the flow of pleasant and unpleasant sensations, this aliveness, this basic knowing of life unfolding, the immediacy of being here, is the ground of our experience.

How does your experience change as you come more into contact with this awareness? You don't have to do anything for bodily life to function, there is nothing to force or control, nothing to demand or defend against. This grounding in your direct experience is an invitation to be where you are, how you are, to let your life be here. Simply. Fully. Freely.

You practise yoga postures, and you may study yoga teachings. But the essence of yoga is this internalisation of your attention; to re-unite yourself with your life. To be inside every posture, to inhabit each breath, emotion, movement; to be truly intimate with life as it unfolds with and around you.

This is the truly transformative aspect of yoga. You are not just transforming your fitness, or your suppleness or your health. You are transforming your life.
It is in this embodied awareness that we find that yoga is union. The way back for Mr Duffy, as for all of us, is to gently inhabit this body. It's where you live.

"Whatever yoga tradition we may practise in, the fundamental ground of yoga, prior to posture and breath, and certainly more primary than how far we stretch or how toned we are, is this direct contact with bodily life."

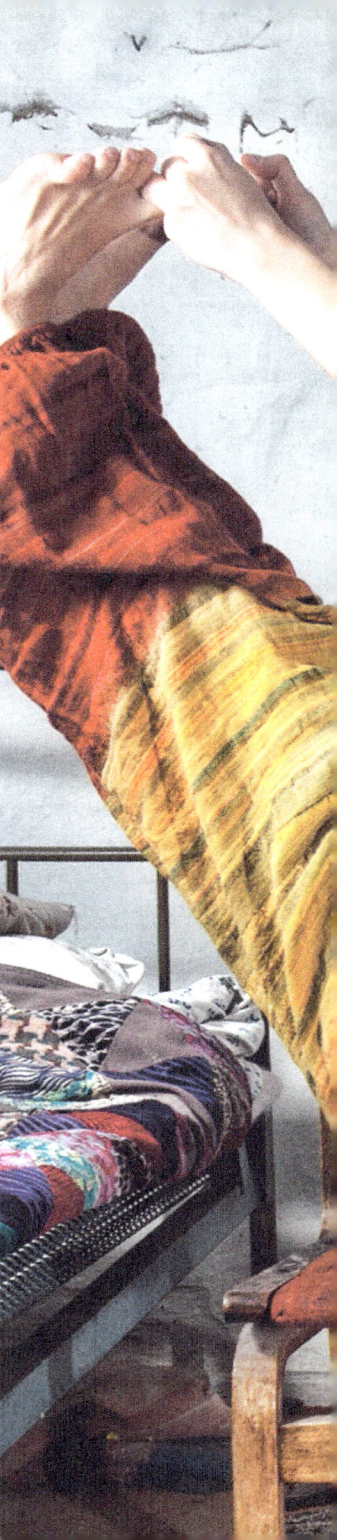

BODHI TREE – Wood

It was under a bodhi tree that the Buddha sat in meditation until he reached enlightenment. This sacred fig tree is a symbol of wisdom, of the ultimate potential that lies within all of us. Its heart-shaped leaves shine the bright green of spring while its bark holds the darkness of the forest; its fruits of knowledge are for everyone who truly desires them. The tree is rooted in the ground and its branches reach towards the heavens, just like human beings are rooted in the material but are pulled in the opposite direction in their search for freedom. One direction represents comfort and the known; the other represents freedom and the unknown. When we practise meditation, we come to realise that nothing is solid or fixed, that everything is in a constant state of flux, and in this knowledge we find the courage to step into the unknown and into freedom.

March 2014

March 2014

					1	2
3	4	5	6	7	8	9
10	11	12	13	14	15	16
17	18	19	20	21	22	23
24	25	26	27	28	29	30
31						

March 2014

3
MONDAY

4
TUESDAY

5
WEDNESDAY

Sutra III.9 *vyutthana nirodha samskarayor abhibhava pradur-*
bhavau nirodha ksana cittanvayo nirodah parinamah

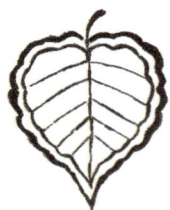

6
THURSDAY

7
FRIDAY

First Quarter 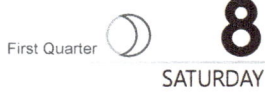 **8**
SATURDAY

9
SUNDAY

March 2014

					1	2	
3	4	5	6	7	8	9	week 10
10	11	12	13	14	15	16	
17	18	19	20	21	22	23	
24	25	26	27	28	29	30	
31							

March 2014

10
MONDAY

11
TUESDAY

12
WEDNESDAY

Sutra III.10 *tasya prasanta vahita samskarat*

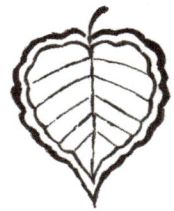

13
THURSDAY

14
FRIDAY

15
SATURDAY

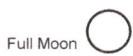Full Moon **16**
SUNDAY

March 2014

						1	2
3	4	5	6	7	8	9
10	11	12	13	14	15	16
17	18	19	20	21	22	23
24	25	26	27	28	29	30
31

week 11

March 2014

17
MONDAY

18
TUESDAY

19
WEDNESDAY

Sutra III.11 *sarvarthataikagratayoh ksyayodayau cittasya samadhiparinamah*

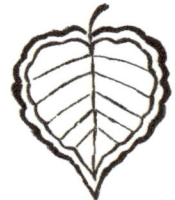

20
Spring Equinox   THURSDAY

21
FRIDAY

22
SATURDAY

23
SUNDAY

March 2014

					1	2
3	4	5	6	7	8	9
10	11	12	13	14	15	16
17	18	19	20	21	22	23
24	25	26	27	28	29	30
31						

week 12

March 2014

24
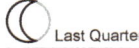 Last Quarter
MONDAY

25
TUESDAY

26
WEDNESDAY

Sutra III.12 *santoditau tulyapratyayau cittasyaikagrata-
parinamah*

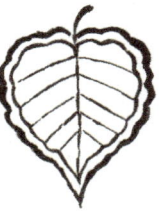

27
THURSDAY

28
FRIDAY

29
SATURDAY

New Moon ○ **30**
SUNDAY

March 2014

					1	2
3	4	5	6	7	8	9
10	11	12	13	14	15	16
17	18	19	20	21	22	23
24	25	26	27	28	29	30
31						

week 13

STIRRUP
Liver Meridian

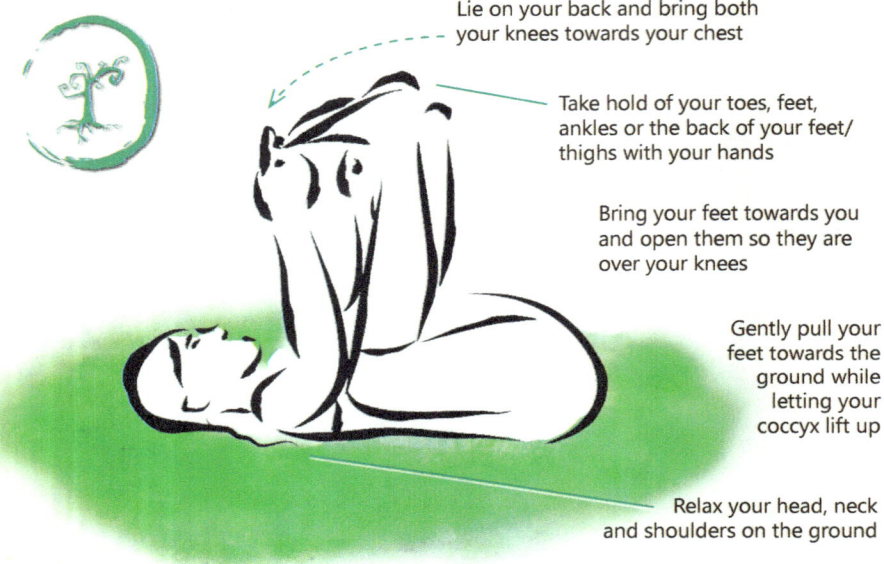

Lie on your back and bring both your knees towards your chest

Take hold of your toes, feet, ankles or the back of your feet/thighs with your hands

Bring your feet towards you and open them so they are over your knees

Gently pull your feet towards the ground while letting your coccyx lift up

Relax your head, neck and shoulders on the ground

While in the Pose

- Holding time: 3 to 5 minutes.
- Breathe deeply and mindfully.

Coming out of the Pose

- Leave the pose slowly and mindfully.
- Exhale and release your feet, draw your knees into your chest and hug your lower legs.
- Observe the effects of the pose.

Modifications and Variations

- If you are tight in your hips use a belt to hold your feet, or do the pose with your feet flat against a wall.
- Bring your feet closer to your buttocks if you feel too much compression in your groins.
- Hold one foot and relax your opposite leg, straight, on the ground. Repeat on the other side.

Taking it Further

- Bring your toes together and pull them closer to your groins, then your chest, then your nose, and finally behind your head.

Meridians and Organs Affected

The Liver, Spleen and Kidney meridians (groins and inner legs).
The Urinary Bladder meridian (dorsal and lumbar spine).
It applies healthy stress to the abdominal organs.

Anatomical Benefits

It deeply opens up the hips.
It strengthens the biceps.
It decompresses and releases the lower back.

Contraindications

This pose is a mild inversion and should be avoided if your blood pressure is very high.
Support your head on a towel or blanket if suffering from neck injury.
Not recommended during pregnancy.

Yang Sibling

Ananda Balasana (Happy Baby Pose). In the Yang yoga version of this pose, we aim to keep the tailbone close to the ground so the lumbar area of the spine and sacrum rest on the ground.

If you feel any painful sensation in your groins, use a variation of the pose!

MY NOTES

Meditation:
A PRACTICAL PERSPECTIVE

By Swami Saradananda

At some point in your life, you have probably experienced meditation. It is not an unnatural thing that only some people can do – meditation is a universal experience, an experience of absolute peace.

People often meditate, even if they don't know they are doing so. To put this into perspective, think of something that you really like to do. Perhaps gardening is your "thing". If so, you can get out there and work for hours without getting tired. It seems that time ceases to exist; you feel very peaceful and happy. This can be seen as a low-level meditation because you still need something outside of yourself to have this experience. Imagine your happy, focused experience intensified many times with your mind becoming so one-pointed that you feel as though you are in total harmony with your experience. This is meditation, an experience of absolute peace.

SOME PRACTICAL POINTS

If you lived in tune with nature, the most effective times for meditation would be dawn and dusk when the atmosphere is charged with a special

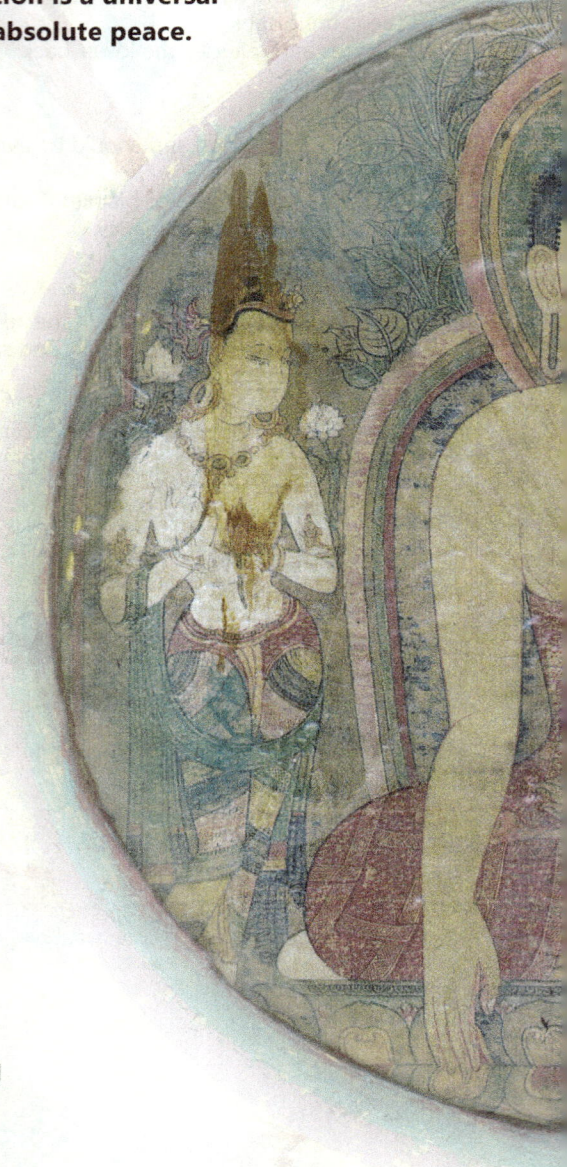

spiritual force. Sunrise and sunset are the most peaceful times of day. Unfortunately, modern lifestyles can make it difficult to practise at dawn and/or at dusk. So, choose a time when you are not involved with other activities and your mind is apt to be calm. This may be early morning, when your mind is still in a pure state and hasn't yet become involved with the work of the day. Or it could be the last thing at night when you can put aside the cares of the day and take the opportunity to tune inwards. Practising at night is like cleansing your mind before sleep. Instead of spending hours tossing, turning and dreaming – which actually uses energy – you quickly fall into a deep restful sleep and wake up in the morning feeling refreshed and energised.

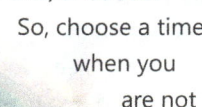

One suggestion is to try to meditate at the same time each day. As your mind will come to associate these times with meditation, it will facilitate the practice itself.

Try to not eat for at least two hours before practising meditation. If you plan to meditate in the early morning hours, make your evening meal a light one.

Decide in advance how long you will sit for meditation. Be determined, no matter what, that you will sit for this period of time. You can set an alarm if you like; there are now many meditation-friendly alarm apps for your phone. Begin with 20 to 30 minutes. Most people find that by meditating for half an hour daily they are able to face life with a peaceful mind and a great resource of inner strength.

> **"Practising at night is like cleansing your mind before sleep. Instead of spending hours tossing, turning and dreaming — which actually uses energy — you quickly fall into a deep restful sleep and wake up in the morning feeling refreshed and energised."**

HOW TO SIT

Sitting in a cross-legged position will greatly facilitate your inward focus, as it helps to physically contain your energy. Your legs form a type of infinity symbol and the pose provides you with a stable, grounded position. To keep your back straight, you may need to sit on a cushion or a rolled-up blanket.

If you are unable to sit cross-legged, kneeling (as in Zen meditation) is an alternative. Sitting in a straight-backed chair is a third alternative, if you have severe physical problems or cannot sit on the floor. If using a chair, make sure to keep your feet flat on the floor and don't cross your ankles.

Whichever position you prefer, make sure that it is a stable one. Remember that every time your body moves, your mind moves. To quiet your mind, begin by quieting your body. Keep your back straight so the energy can travel up your spine and your breath can be full. Take slow, deep breaths to ensure that a liberal supply of oxygen reaches your brain. You may find it helpful to imagine a string drawing your head skywards – and a second thread attached to your breastbone so that your lungs have sufficient space to expand fully.

Close your eyes and bring your awareness on your breath. Don't try to control your breath, just watch it. Joyously draw in life with each inhalation. Release pent-up emotions and impurities with each exhalation. Gradually your mind will become calm.

Don't put off starting your meditation practice; start today and practise daily.

MY NOTES

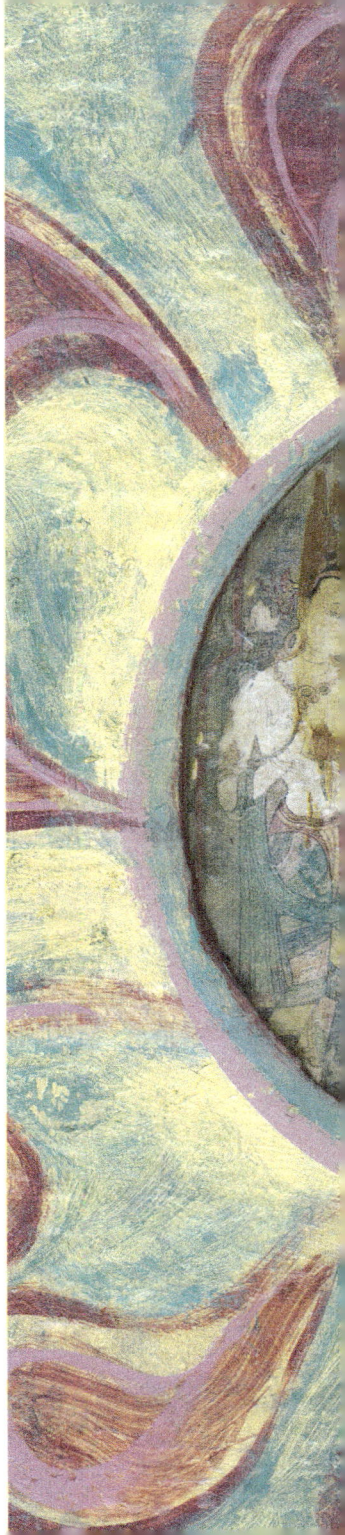

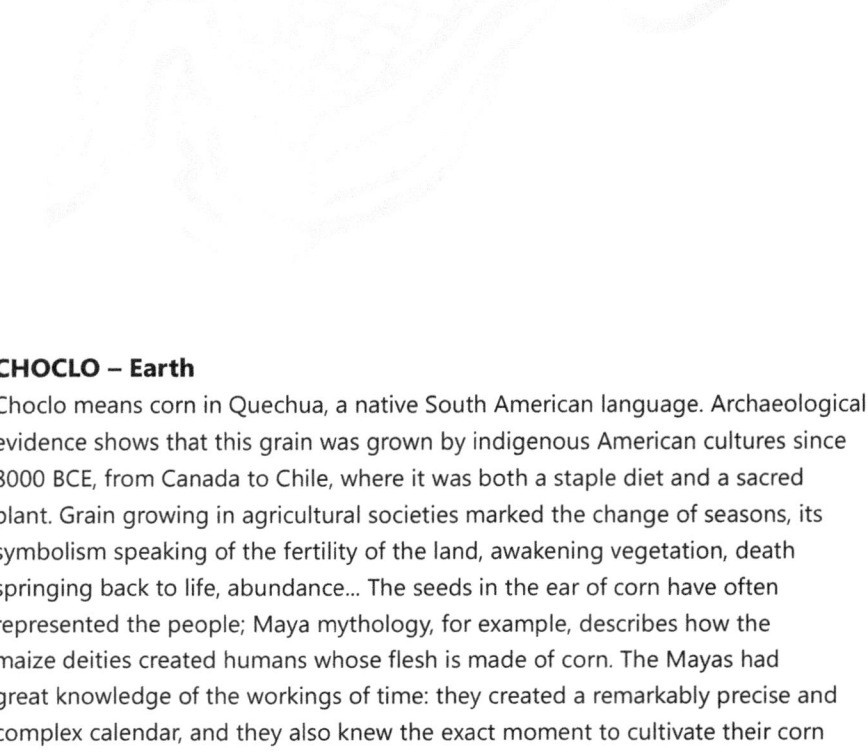

CHOCLO – Earth

Choclo means corn in Quechua, a native South American language. Archaeological evidence shows that this grain was grown by indigenous American cultures since 8000 BCE, from Canada to Chile, where it was both a staple diet and a sacred plant. Grain growing in agricultural societies marked the change of seasons, its symbolism speaking of the fertility of the land, awakening vegetation, death springing back to life, abundance... The seeds in the ear of corn have often represented the people; Maya mythology, for example, describes how the maize deities created humans whose flesh is made of corn. The Mayas had great knowledge of the workings of time: they created a remarkably precise and complex calendar, and they also knew the exact moment to cultivate their corn to generate abundance. Can we too learn to respect the right timing that brings about abundance in different areas of our lives?

April 2014

April 2014

	1	2	3	4	5	6
7	8	9	10	11	12	13
14	15	16	17	18	19	20
21	22	23	24	25	26	27
28	29	30				

31
MONDAY

1
TUESDAY

2
WEDNESDAY

Sutra III.13 *etena bhutendriyesu dharma laksanavastha parinama vyakhyatah*

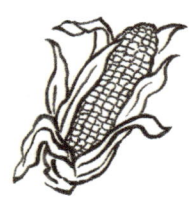

3
THURSDAY

4
FRIDAY

5
SATURDAY

6
SUNDAY

April 2014

	1	2	3	4	5	6	week 14
7	8	9	10	11	12	13	
14	15	16	17	18	19	20	
21	22	23	24	25	26	27	
28	29	30					

7 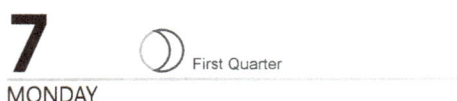 First Quarter
MONDAY

8
TUESDAY

9
WEDNESDAY

Sutra III.14 *santoditavyapadesya dharmanupati dharmi*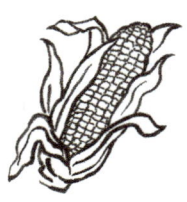

April 2014

10
THURSDAY

11
FRIDAY

12
SATURDAY

13
SUNDAY

April 2014

	1	2	3	4	5	6
7	8	9	10	11	12	13
14	15	16	17	18	19	20
21	22	23	24	25	26	27
28	29	30				

week 15

April 2014

14
MONDAY

15
TUESDAY

 Full Moon

Total Lunar Eclipse

16
WEDNESDAY

Sutra III.15 *kramanyatvam parinamanyatve hetuh*

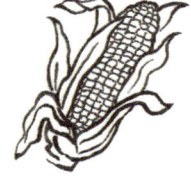

17
THURSDAY

18 FRIDAY

19
SATURDAY

20 SUNDAY

April 2014

	1	2	3	4	5	6
7	8	9	10	11	12	13
14	15	16	17	18	19	20
21	22	23	24	25	26	27
28	29	30				

week 16

21
MONDAY

22 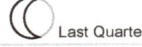 Last Quarter
TUESDAY

23
WEDNESDAY

Sutra III.16 *parinama traya samyamad atitanagata jnanam*

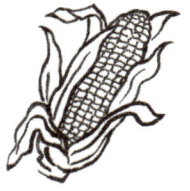

24
THURSDAY

25
FRIDAY

26
SATURDAY

27
SUNDAY

April 2014

	1	2	3	4	5	6
7	8	9	10	11	12	13
14	15	16	17	18	19	20
21	22	23	24	25	26	27
28	29	30				

week 17

April 2014

28
MONDAY

29
TUESDAY

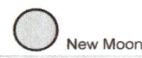 New Moon

Annular Solar Eclipse

30
WEDNESDAY

Sutra III.17 *sabdartha pratyayanam itaretaradhyasat samkaras tat pravibhaga samyamat sarva bhuta ruta jnanam*

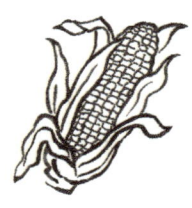

1
THURSDAY

2
FRIDAY

3
SATURDAY

4
SUNDAY

April 2014

	1	2	3	4	5	6
7	8	9	10	11	12	13
14	15	16	17	18	19	20
21	22	23	24	25	26	27
28	29	30				

week 18

SQUARE
Liver Meridian

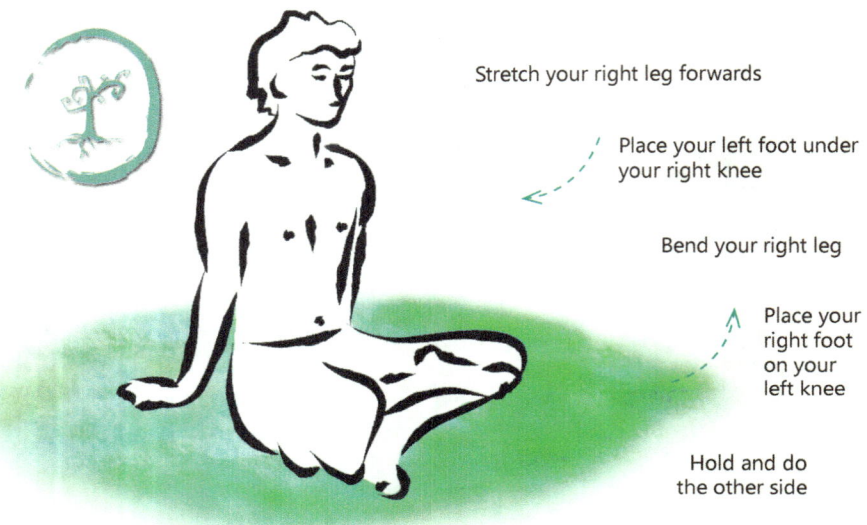

Stretch your right leg forwards

Place your left foot under your right knee

Bend your right leg

Place your right foot on your left knee

Hold and do the other side

While in the Pose

- Holding time: 3 to 5 minutes on each side.
- Breathe deeply and mindfully.

Coming out of the Pose

- Leave the pose slowly and mindfully.
- On an inhalation, lean slightly back while resting on your hands.
- Stretch your legs in front of you and allow your knees to release any tension.
- Observe the effects of the pose.

Modifications and Variations

- If you experience pain in your knees feel free to place your feet in front of or on the outside of your knees (rather than on top of or below them).
- If you suffer from sciatica, sit on a cushion to elevate your hips higher than your knees.
- For tight hips: lie on your back and place your right foot against a wall (leg making an approximately 90 degree angle). Bend your left leg and place your left ankle on your right thigh. To make it stronger, slide the right foot down the wall.

Taking it Further

- Make a perfect square with your legs and bend forwards to intensify the stress on your hips.

Meridians and Organs Affected

The Liver and Kidney meridians (groins and inner legs).
The Gall Bladder meridian (outer legs).
It massages the ovaries (when bending forwards).

Anatomical Benefits

It deeply opens up the hips.
It releases the lumbar spine (when bending forwards).

Contraindications

Knee issues.
Very tight hips.
Severe sciatica problems.

Yang Sibling

Agnistambhasana (Fire Log Pose). In the Yang yoga variation of this pose, the torso is actively lifting up towards the sky while the feet are flexed to keep the leg muscles engaged.

If you feel any painful sensation in your knees, use a variation of the pose!

MY NOTES

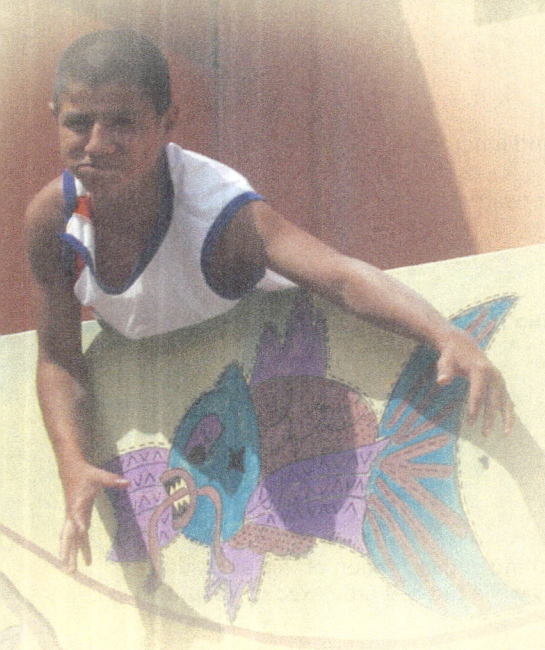

Yoga Beyond The Mat:
THE CHOCLO PROJECT

By Elena Sepúlveda

Choclo is a Quechua word for corn, a plant that has been a staple diet in Andean and other Latin American cultures for centuries. It's also the name for a project that brings together underprivileged children in Peru and yoga clothing in a highly creative and ethical way.

For a corn (and colour!) lover like me, coming across the Choclo Project clothing was a very enjoyable surprise. Their beautiful prints and original designs caught my attention instantly the first time I saw them. I remember it was a very windy day in Barcelona and their hoodies, pants, tops, etc. seemed to be alive on their railings at the brand's stand during a Barcelona Yoga Conference. Choclo Project? What kind of project could this possibly be? I had to know!

It turned out that behind these gorgeous and versatile garments, there was a story. "If you have ever been touched by the image of a smiling child living in total poverty then you may understand where we are coming from, because it was this very experience that planted the seed that would grow into the Choclo Project", explains Roland Wimbush, founder of the Choclo Project. And the seed did grow... The brand has been sponsoring the non-profit orphanage Nuevo Futuro in Lima, Peru, since 2009. "The purchase of one Debi hoodie, for example, equates to some generic Panadol for a fever or a papaya fruit or 2 litres of milk. Our goal is to keep growing so we are able to improve the lives of more children and provide them with a safe and creative environment," adds Roland.

Each Choclo Project product displays either a discreet or more visible artwork inspired by a drawing by one of the children in the brand's partner associations. To design their SS14 collection, they went to the little surf town of

Huanchaco, also in Peru, where they lived, created and surfed with the ex-street kids from Mundo de Niños for two months. Their goal was to nourish the children's natural talent by teaching them new techniques that helped them express themselves

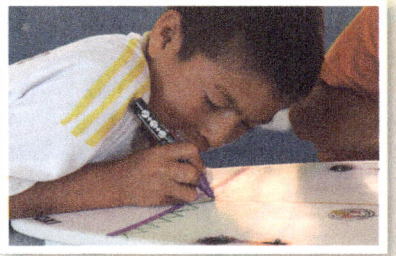

creatively. During this time, they hosted workshops in which the participants drew, cut paper, created animations, decorated a surfboard and painted a large outdoor mural. "The most important thing, even more important than the donation," says Roland, "is the feeling of importance it gives the kids knowing that their imagination has real value."

"It was a pretty amazing experience in so many ways even though it took some time for us to convince the children that

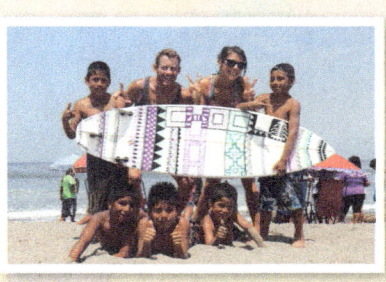

what they drew really didn't matter as long as they were expressing themselves and having fun. Once they understood this, things really got interesting. The highlight was probably the last evening once we had finished the mural. The children and the tutors organised a bonfire for us on the beach. Each of the children said a few words about what they had got out of the projects and the two months we had spent together. We also said a few words to thank them all for their efforts and enthusiasm. It was very emotional and even though we know we will be back soon we miss them a lot."

"The 2014 collection is inspired by Peru as a whole. Most of the creative projects we did with the children involved working with simple geometric forms and creating patterns such as the artwork on the surfboard. We then used these elements to create ethnic style motifs and shapes that are very simple and pure. The range is as fresh as ever, drawing inspiration from the colours of the local markets we frequented and the extreme landscape that surrounded us. Peru also has a very rich textile culture and particularly in organic cotton. We went and met the farmers in Chincha and listened intently as they explained how they farm organically and how they democratically manage the irrigation system of their own land using water flowing into the valley naturally from the mountains. We are really happy to be able to support these farmers by producing a part of the 2014 collection in Peru. We are aiming to produce 100% of our 2014 product range in organic fabric, which has been a major goal for us since we launched the brand."

"If you have ever been touched by the image of a smiling child living in total poverty then you may understand where we are coming from."

The Choclo Project is also working with UK-based Amantani. This NGO works to bridge the gap between home and school for kids living in Ccorca, a small Quechua district in the Southern Peruvian Andes, where children have to walk very long distances to attend school. After visiting their boarding houses in 2013, they decided to team up and make some limited edition T-shirts with photos taken by the children with disposable cameras – as part of the NGO's Meet My World Photography Competition. As with all other Choclo Project products, 5% of the sale price goes to Amantani.

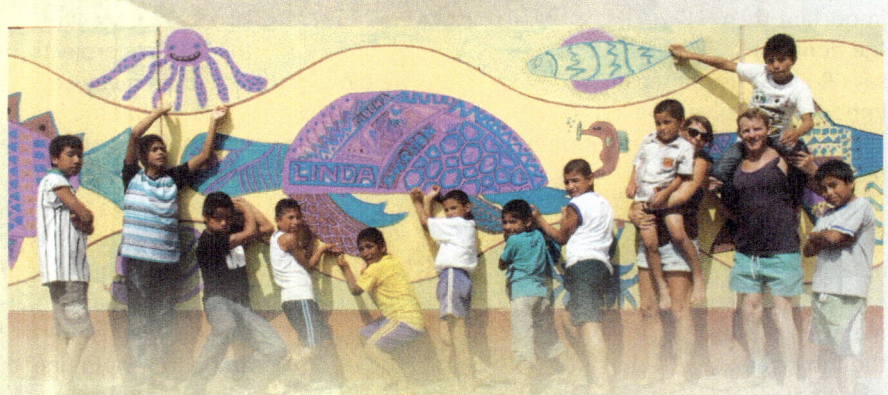

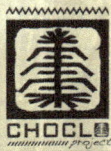

To know more about this project, its work with the kids in Peru and its clothing, visit their website:
www.ChocloProject.com
or http://www.facebook.com/ChocloProjectClothing

MY NOTES

CLOVER – Wood

In the very early days Celtic people believed that if you carried a shamrock, or three-leaf clover, it was possible to see evil spirits approaching; four-leaf clovers were said to offer magical protection, to ward off bad luck and to mantle the carrier in a cloak of good fortune. Today, because they grow so quickly and in such large numbers, clover is considered by many a symbol of energy and vitality. But only the four-leaf variety is said to be bring good luck to those who come across it. Lucky symbols in all cultures are as bountiful as clover in the fields during spring: a horseshoe, the number "7", a rainbow, a ladybird or a wishbone may be some we are familiar with. When we believe in them, even for one split second, we align our minds with potential happy events. Perhaps it is then when the magic occurs?

May 2014

JOURNAL

May 2014

			1	2	3	4
5	6	7	8	9	10	11
12	13	14	15	16	17	18
19	20	21	22	23	24	25
26	27	28	29	30	31	

5
MONDAY

6
TUESDAY

7
 First Quarter
WEDNESDAY

Sutra III.18 *samskara saksatkaranat purva jatijnanam*

8
THURSDAY

9
FRIDAY

10
SATURDAY

11
SUNDAY

May 2014

			1	2	3	4
5	6	7	8	9	10	11
12	13	14	15	16	17	18
19	20	21	22	23	24	25
26	27	28	29	30	31	

week 19

12
MONDAY

13
TUESDAY

14 Full Moon
WEDNESDAY

Sutra III.19 *pratyayasya parachitta jnanam*

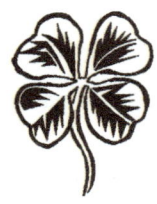

15
THURSDAY

16
FRIDAY

17
SATURDAY

18
SUNDAY

May 2014

			1	2	3	4
5	6	7	8	9	10	11
12	13	14	15	16	17	18
19	20	21	22	23	24	25
26	27	28	29	30	31	

week 20

19
MONDAY

20
TUESDAY

21
WEDNESDAY

◖ Last Quarter

Sutra III.20 *na ca tat salambanam tasyavisayi bhutatvat*

22
THURSDAY

23
FRIDAY

24
SATURDAY

25
SUNDAY

May 2014

			1	2	3	4
5	6	7	8	9	10	11
12	13	14	15	16	17	18
19	20	21	22	23	24	25
26	27	28	29	30	31	

week 21

May 2014

26
MONDAY

27
TUESDAY

28
⊙ New Moon
WEDNESDAY

Sutra III.21 *kayarupa samyamat tadgrahya sakti stambhe caksuh prakasasamprayoge ntardhanam*

29
THURSDAY

30
FRIDAY

31
SATURDAY

1
SUNDAY

May 2014

			1	2	3	4
5	6	7	8	9	10	11
12	13	14	15	16	17	18
19	20	21	22	23	24	25
26	27	28	29	30	31	

week 22

BUTTERFLY
Gall Bladder Meridian

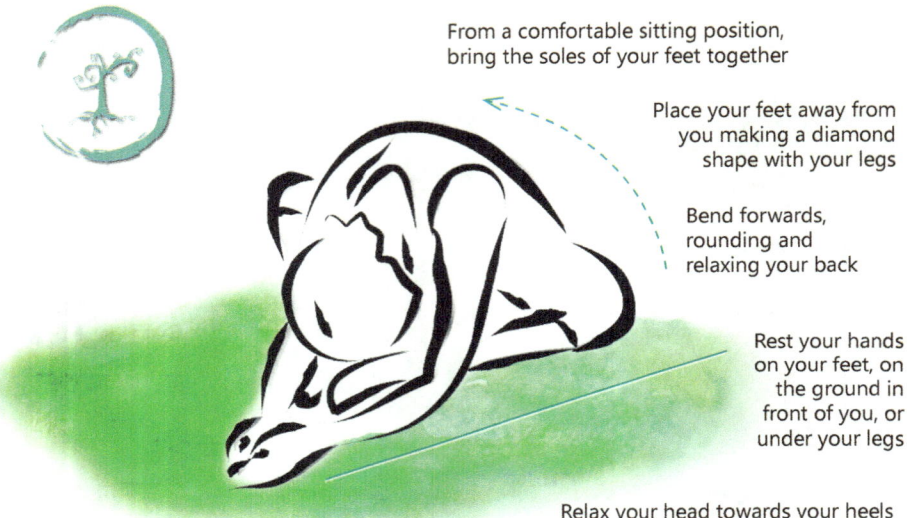

From a comfortable sitting position, bring the soles of your feet together

Place your feet away from you making a diamond shape with your legs

Bend forwards, rounding and relaxing your back

Rest your hands on your feet, on the ground in front of you, or under your legs

Relax your head towards your heels

While in the Pose

- Holding time: 3 minutes or much longer.
- Breathe deeply and mindfully.

Coming out of the Pose

- Leave the pose slowly and mindfully.
- Inhale and slowly come back to an upright position. Stretch your legs forwards. Place your hands on the ground next to your hips with your arms extended and rest back creating a very mild back bend.
- Observe the effects of the pose.

Modifications and Variations

- If you suffer from sciatica, try placing a cushion under your buttocks to elevate your hips higher than your knees, helping your hips to rotate forwards.
- Move your feet further away if your lower back or inner thighs feel tight.
- Support your head on your hands or a cushion if you start to build up tension in your neck or head.

Taking it Further

- Let the weight of your upper body sink further into the ground with each exhalation.
- Bring your arms under your legs or relax them behind your body.

Meridians and Organs Affected

The Gall Bladder meridian (outer legs).
The Urinary Bladder meridian (lumbar and dorsal spine).
The Kidney and Liver meridians (inner legs and groins).
It creates healthy stress on the ovaries.

Anatomical Benefits

It stretches the lower back.
When the feet are further away from the groins, it stretches the backs of the thighs.
When the feet are closer to the groins, it stretches the insides of the thighs.
It creates healthy stress on the ovaries.

Contraindications

It can aggravate sciatica.
Avoid if the neck has a reverse curvature.

Yang Sibling

Baddha Konasana (Bound Angle Pose). In the Yang yoga version of this pose, the spine is kept straight and the feet are closer to the groins.

If you feel any painful sensation in your neck or sacral area, use a variation of the pose!

MY NOTES

Yin & Yang Yoga:
THE PERFECT COMBO

By José de Groot

Yin Yoga is hot! More and more yogis are getting "hooked" on this quiet, intense and meditative practice. Many people come to their first Yin class not knowing what to expect, but most of them are (pleasantly) surprised by the power of Yin.

But let me start by explaining what the essential difference is between Yin and Yang yoga. It is useful to know that the terms yin and yang come from the Chinese Daoist view, where yang represents the active, dynamic elements of life, and yin the passive and introspective.

Keep in mind that Yin yoga can be best described as a deep and meditative practice that enhances your awareness, allows you to feel more subtle energies and sensations, and it teaches you to relax profoundly. It prepares the mind and body for long meditation sessions and stimulates the vital energy (chi) that flows through the fascia (where the meridians are situated), nurturing, balancing and healing your physical, emotional and mental well-being.

"Yang yoga" on the other hand is a term used to refer to all dynamic styles of yoga such as: Hatha, Vinyasa, Ashtanga, Power, etc. The goal of these types of yoga is to build internal heat using Ujjayi breathing and dynamic sequences consisting of repeated asanas which strengthen, lengthen and tone primarily the muscles of your body. It also enhances your digestion, deepens your breath and relaxes your mind.

So in short, Yang yoga targets muscle and Yin yoga targets fascia. In order for you to work out your muscles in Yang yoga you need rhythmic and repetitive movement. In doing so, you will feel more energetic, muscularly flexible, stronger and less tense. In Yin yoga you stimulate the deeper tissues of your body, called fascia. As these tissues are more rigid, they need a different approach than the more elastic tissues of our bodies (like muscles). So, in your Yin practice your aim is to be still in the pose and hold it for a period of five minutes or more, trying to relax instead of engaging the muscles. In doing so, the fascia is being targeted.

But what is fascia exactly? Fascia is like a net or matrix that holds everything we are together. Your whole body make up is a continuum of fascia expressed in different forms, density and function. Fascia exists, for example, within and around the muscle (mio-fascia), in its more dense form it is called a tendon, ligament, joint-capsule, cartilage or bone. Yin yoga targets all forms of the fascia, and as a result you regain and/or expand its original range of motion. You will feel more open and flexible especially in the pelvis, your whole back and hips. To know more about fascia, see pp. 172-174.

Even though Yin and Yang yoga are different styles, they complement each other in reaching their common goal: to purify balance and harmonise our bodies and minds. But most of all they enable us to tune in with our true nature so that the energy within and around us can flow freely.

It is essential to remember that no two bodies are alike; the size, weight, form of your bones, organs, muscles, nerves etc are unique. There is no one in this world exactly like you. In particular, your skeletal structure determines when you have opened up your tissues enough, how you move and why you can or can't do a certain yoga pose. So in choosing your yoga practice, either Yin or Yang or a mix, the key part is to develop awareness which helps you to observe your daily needs (mentally, emotionally and physically) so you can adapt your yoga practice to them. In doing so your practice will be balanced out, personal, therapeutic and a lot more fun!

The growing popularity of Yin yoga comes from a realisation that some types of "Yang" yoga practices are a reflection of our very yang style of living. They enhance the yang energy even more, creating more imbalance instead of coming closer to the peaceful coexistence of activity (yang) and passivity (yin).

"In choosing your yoga practice, either Yin or Yang or a mix, the key part is to develop awareness which helps you to observe your daily needs (mentally, emotionally and physically) so you can adapt your yoga practice to them."

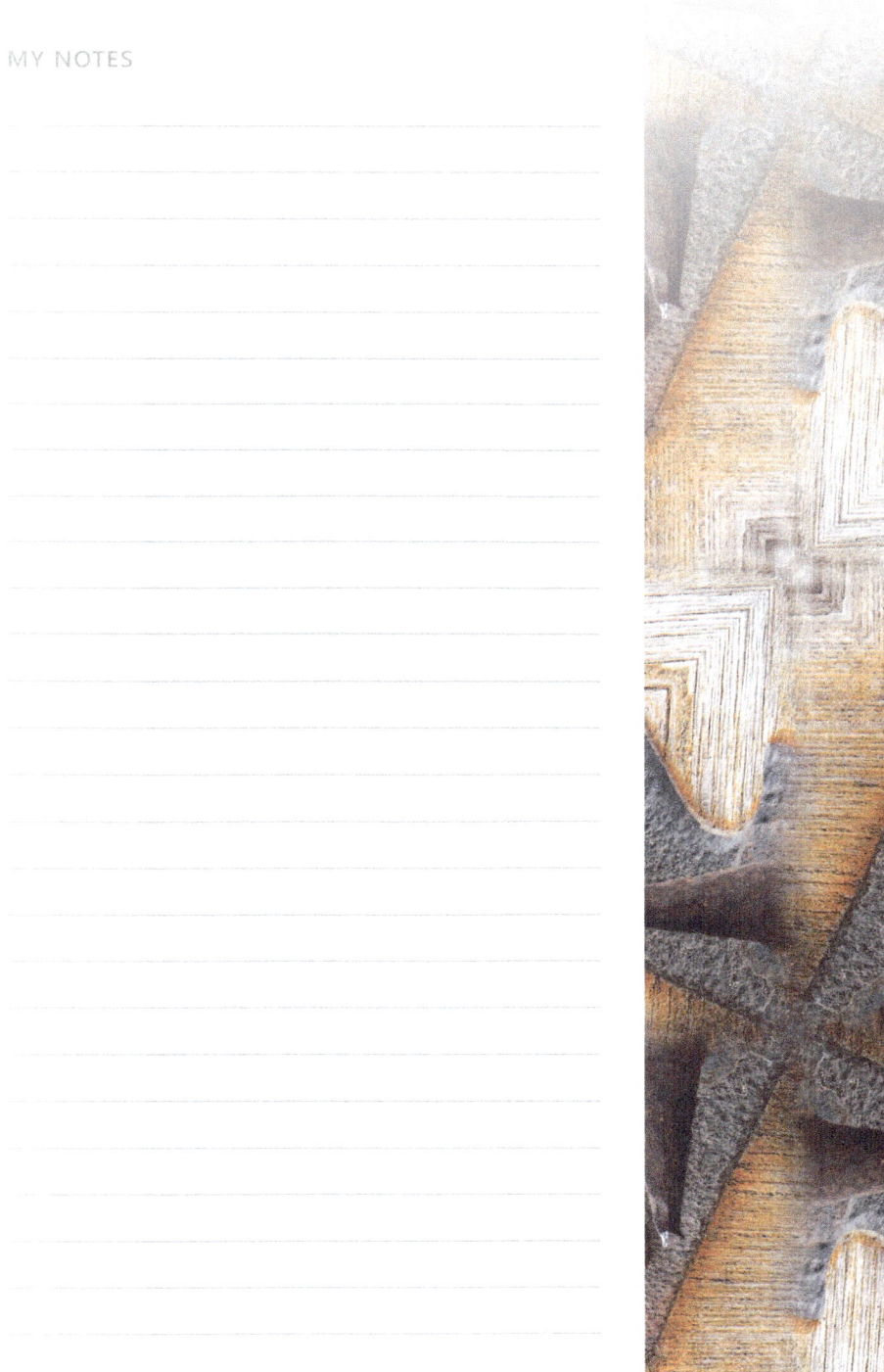

AGNI – Fire

Fire has ambivalent qualities. Either divine or demonic, creative or destructive, revered or feared, it is a primal universal symbol said to have the power to devour things and return them to their original purity. In Hinduism, the god of fire Agni has 10 different forms. One of them is the "digestive fire", which according to the ancient science of Ayurveda, is responsible for absorbing the nutrients needed by the body while burning off toxic waste products. More broadly, it refers to our capacity to process the different aspects of life: experiences, emotions, memories, sensory impressions, etc. A strong Agni leads to health and well-being, and will serve the absorption and purifying process within body and mind. A weak Agni is a ticket to disease. Yoga has specific practices designed to strengthen and balance our inner Agni. Don't miss out on them!

June 2014

June 2014

						1
2	3	4	5	6	7	8
9	10	11	12	13	14	15
16	17	18	19	20	21	22
23	24	25	26	27	28	29
30						

June 2014

2
MONDAY

3
TUESDAY

4
WEDNESDAY

Sutra III.22 *etena sabdadyantardhanam uktam*

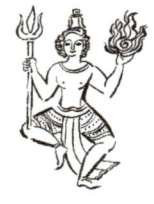

First Quarter

5
THURSDAY

6
FRIDAY

7
SATURDAY

8
SUNDAY

June 2014

						1
2	3	4	5	6	7	8
9	10	11	12	13	14	15
16	17	18	19	20	21	22
23	24	25	26	27	28	29
30						

week 23

June 2014

9
MONDAY

10
TUESDAY

11
WEDNESDAY

Sutra III.23 *sopakramam nirupakraman ca karma tat samyamad aparanta jnanam aristebhyo va*

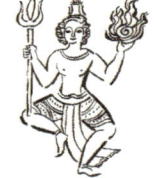

12
THURSDAY

Full Moon ◯ **13**
FRIDAY

14
SATURDAY

15
SUNDAY

June 2014

						1
2	3	4	5	6	7	8
9	10	11	12	13	14	15
16	17	18	19	20	21	22
23	24	25	26	27	28	29
30						

week 24

June 2014

16
MONDAY

17
TUESDAY

18
WEDNESDAY

Sutra III.24 *maitryadisu balani*

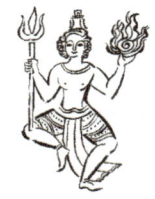

Last Quarter ☾ **19**
THURSDAY

20
FRIDAY

Summer Solstice **21**
SATURDAY

22
SUNDAY

June 2014

						1
2	3	4	5	6	7	8
9	10	11	12	13	14	15
16	17	18	19	20	21	22
23	24	25	26	27	28	29
30						

week 25

June 2014

23
MONDAY

24
TUESDAY

25
WEDNESDAY

Sutra III.25 *balesu hasti baladini*

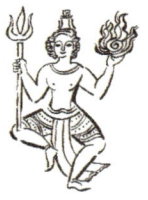

26
THURSDAY

New Moon ◯ **27**
FRIDAY

28
SATURDAY

29
SUNDAY

June 2014

						1
2	3	4	5	6	7	8
9	10	11	12	13	14	15
16	17	18	19	20	21	22
23	24	25	26	27	28	29
30						

week 26

ANAHATASANA
Heart Meridian

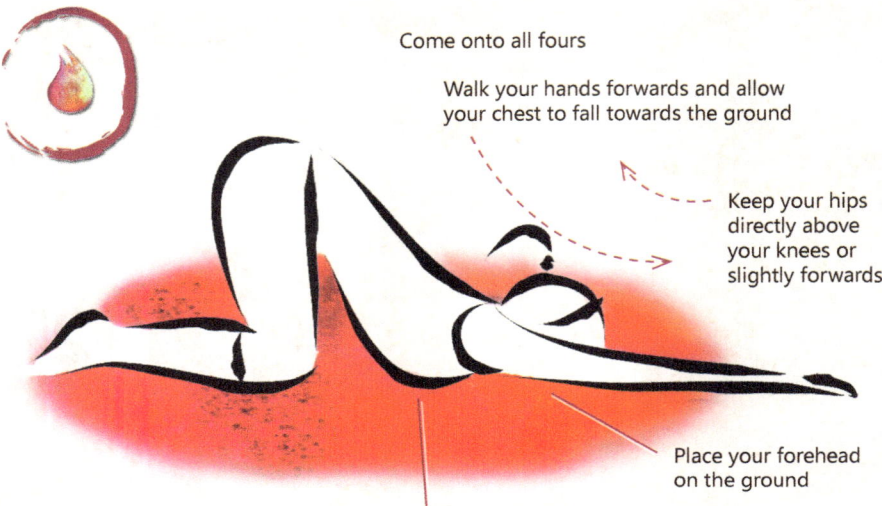

Come onto all fours

Walk your hands forwards and allow your chest to fall towards the ground

Keep your hips directly above your knees or slightly forwards

Place your forehead on the ground

Let your heart melt into the ground

While in the Pose

- Holding time: 3 to 5 minutes.
- Breathe deeply and mindfully.

Coming out of the Pose

- Leave the pose slowly and mindfully.
- Inhale and slowly walk your hands back towards you. On an exhalation, push the ground with your hands and take your hips towards your heels to rest in Balasana (Child's Pose). Let your arms rest to the sides of your body.
- Observe the effects of the pose.

Modifications and Variations

- If experiencing shoulder pain or numbness in your hands or fingers, experiment with the position of your arms, bending them or moving them apart.
- Rest your forehead or your chest on a bolster.
- Protect your knees with a blanket if necessary.

Taking it Further

- Place your chin instead of your forehead on the ground. This will create further compression on your neck vertebrae, so make sure it is appropriate for you.
- Tuck your toes in to stretch the soles of your feet and compress your ankles.

Meridians and Organs Affected

The Heart and Lung meridians (inner arms).
The Stomach, Kidney and Spleen meridians (front of torso).
It is said to soften the heart.

Anatomical Benefits

It stretches and opens up the throat, shoulders, armpits, chest and belly.

Contraindications

Cervical issues.
Shoulder injuries.

Yang Sibling

Uttana Shishosana (Extended Puppy Pose). In the Yang yoga version of this pose, the arms are active and the shoulders don't touch the ground. The hands are pressing down while the hips are pulling back towards the heels to stretch the spine.

If you feel any painful sensation in your shoulders or neck, use a variation of the pose!

MY NOTES

The Koshas:
UNLEASHING YOGA'S POTENTIAL

By Sarah Dawson

Yoga works on our anatomy; strengthening and stretching the muscles, mobilising the spine and joints and nourishing our internal organs and systems. But there is much more than that happening behind the scenes.

When you undertake a tricky rotated Trikonasana (Triangle Pose), take flight on one leg in Garudasana (Eagle Pose), or gracefully balance in Natarajasana (Lord of the Dance Pose) something deep is taking place beneath the surface.

Each asana is doing much more than simply honing and toning the physique – every posture activates, calms or stimulates the chakras, the body's energy centres, bringing balance and harmony and making yoga an entirely holistic form of exercise.

As well as awareness of the power of the chakras, you can enhance your yoga practice further by being mindful of the body's koshas, the different layers of existence in life, our "subtle" nature. When these are in balance you can experience daivam (a Sanskrit word – the language of the Vedas – which roughly translates to mean enrichment, opportunity and good fortune).

Yoga becomes much more than a physical practice, and ever more enriching when you work with the subtleties of the chakras and koshas to unleash their spiritual and psychic potential. Here's how:

- Akarana Dhanurasana (Standing Archer Pose, performed from Virabhadrasana I or Warrior I) is a fantastic asana to dedicate to a life goal. As you bend then draw your arm behind you (the bow), focus your mind on a dream you would like to fulfil. Keep it pure (in your heart centre) then as you shoot your arrow towards your target, visualise your dream/goal coming to fruition. Repeat, and trust in the power of intention.

- In Ustrasana (Camel Pose), widely arc your arms behind you to rest on your lower back, the back of your thighs, or heels, and visualise drawing a golden light overhead. Breathe this healing light into your heart and lungs, clearsing, healing and unblocking painful emotions. Visualise sadness, loss and grief being dissolved by the golden light, and transformed into peacefulness and acceptance. Working with the koshas in this way (through manomaya and vijnanamaya, as well as the breath and physical koshas) will help to restore balance and harmony.

- Ardha Matsyendrasana (Half Lord of the Fishes Pose) can help feelings of jealousy or insecurity melt away. Breathing deeply and twisting your body to either side raises energy from the root chakra into the heart, via the sacral and solar plexus chakras, allowing creative juices to rise, your personal power to shine, and reminding you of your own glorious uniqueness. So as you twist be aware of the physical movement, your breath making the pose all the sweeter, then tune into your thoughts and feelings. Picture your insecurities and doubts being transformed into generosity by a pink light of love, leaving you with a complete sense of security and confidence in your own skin.

- When balancing on one leg in Garudasana (Eagle Pose) with your arms positioned to resemble its beak, imagine that you are this magnificent bird that carried the Hindu god Vishnu, perched high on a mountain ready to take flight. Cultivate the bird's poise, balance and calm and allow your intuition to open and wisdom to rise. Chances are you'll experience a "light-bulb" moment afterwards as energy rises to the third eye (ajna chakra), via the heart, removing mental fuzziness and confusion.

If you've ever finished your practice "floating on air", it's likely that you've touched daivam. And if you're wondering how to get deep down into the "D factor" as you move into your steady pose or flow in and out of a sequence, bring your awareness into the physical body (annamaya kosha). Then notice your breath – the physiology layer (pranamaya kosha) – allowing your practice to be smoother, effortless, rejuvenating and releasing.

Go deeper by "tuning into" the thought layer (vijnanamaya kosha) and, for example, mentally visualising a glorious bird when performing Garudasana, or a magnificent oak tree when balancing in Vrkasana (Tree Pose), drawing on its qualities.

Then gently, and without judgement, enquire inwardly as to how the pose/flow is making you feel. Now you're accessing your emotional layer (manomaya kosha). Your consciousness will bring you to a very still and tranquil place – the blissful layer (anandamaya kosha) – also known as the Self.

"Yoga becomes much more than a physical practice, and ever more enriching when you work with the subtleties of the chakras and koshas to unleash their spiritual and psychic potential."

MY NOTES

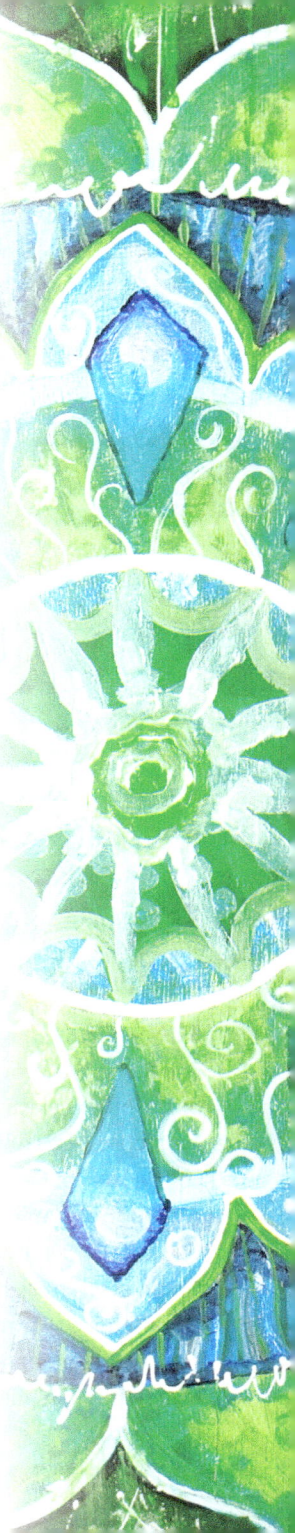

SUN – Fire

The Sun is the central star of our planetary system; it determines the direction of the other celestial bodies and provides certain conditions for life. The sun symbolises the centre, life, vitality, the heart, warmth, knowledge, light... On a smaller scale, the human essence can be seen as a microcosm of that Sun that rises in the morning, reaches a peak, falls into darkness at night and rises the next day. Our lives mirror what we see in the sky in an endless cycle of death and birth. On an even smaller scale, our inner self could be viewed as a Sun that shines our life-affirming warmth onto other human beings. Seeing ourselves as powerful suns can be sobering and humbling: what conditions are we creating for the lives of our loved ones in a universe populated by as many people as there are stars in the sky?

July 2014

July 2014

	1	2	3	4	5	6
7	8	9	10	11	12	13
14	15	16	17	18	19	20
21	22	23	24	25	26	27
28	29	30	31			

June / July 2014

30
MONDAY

1
TUESDAY

2
WEDNESDAY

Sutra III.26 *pravrttyaloka nyasat suksma vyavahita viprakrsta jnanam*

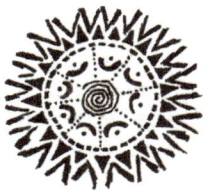

3
THURSDAY

4
FRIDAY

First Quarter ☽ **5**
SATURDAY

6
SUNDAY

July 2014

1	2	3	4	5	6	week 27
7	8	9	10	11	12	13
14	15	16	17	18	19	20
21	22	23	24	25	26	27
28	29	30	31			

July 2014

7
MONDAY

8
TUESDAY

9
WEDNESDAY

Sutra III.27 *bhuvana jnanam surye samyamat*

10
THURSDAY

11
FRIDAY

Full Moon

12
SATURDAY

13
SUNDAY

July 2014

	1	2	3	4	5	6	
7	8	9	10	11	12	13	week 28
14	15	16	17	18	19	20	
21	22	23	24	25	26	27	
28	29	30	31				

14
MONDAY

15
TUESDAY

16
WEDNESDAY

Sutra III.28 *candre tara vyuha jnanam*

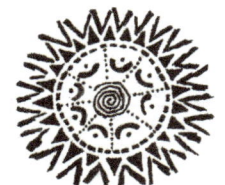

17
THURSDAY

18
FRIDAY

Last Quarter 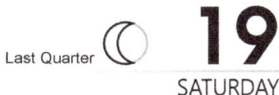 19
SATURDAY

20
SUNDAY

July 2014

	1	2	3	4	5	6
7	8	9	10	11	12	13
14	15	16	17	18	19	20	week 29
21	22	23	24	25	26	27
28	29	30	31			

21
MONDAY

22
TUESDAY

23
WEDNESDAY

Sutra III.29 *dhurve tadgati jnanam*

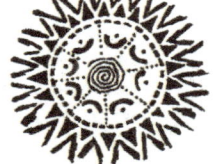

24
THURSDAY

25
FRIDAY

New Moon ◯ **26**
SATURDAY

27
SUNDAY

July 2014

	1	2	3	4	5	6
7	8	9	10	11	12	13
14	15	16	17	18	19	20
21	22	23	24	25	26	27
28	29	30	31			

week 30

July 2014

28
MONDAY

29
TUESDAY

30
WEDNESDAY

Sutra III.30 *nabhi cakre kaya vyuha jnanam*

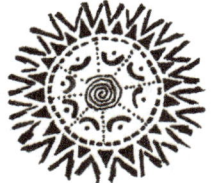

31
THURSDAY

1
FRIDAY

2
SATURDAY

3
SUNDAY

July 2014

	1	2	3	4	5	6
7	8	9	10	11	12	13
14	15	16	17	18	19	20
21	22	23	24	25	26	27
28	29	30	31			

week 31

RECLINING TWIST
Small Intestine Meridian

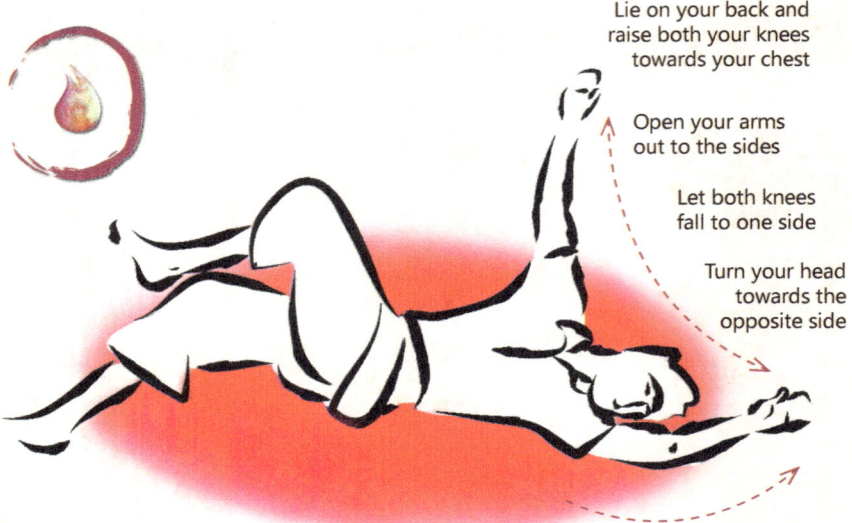

Lie on your back and raise both your knees towards your chest

Open your arms out to the sides

Let both knees fall to one side

Turn your head towards the opposite side

Raise your arm on the same side you are facing to find a stretch along your chest

While in the Pose

- Holding time: 3 to 5 minutes on each side.
- Breathe deeply and mindfully.

Coming out of the Pose

- Leave the pose slowly and mindfully.
- On an inhalation, return your knees to the centre. Hug them into your chest while gently rocking from side to side.
- Observe the effects of the pose.

Modifications and Variations

- If you feel any numbness or a tingling sensation in your hand or arm, bend the outstretched arm, place it on a cushion or even take it down.
- Cross your knees before letting them fall to the side.

Taking it Further

- Stretch the top leg on the ground bringing it towards your face to stretch your glutes and outer leg.
- Take hold of the foot of your bottom leg with the opposite hand and pull it towards you to further compress the lumbar area and stretch that thigh.

Meridians and Organs Affected

The Heart, Lung and Small Intestine meridian (outer and inner arm).
The Urinary Bladder meridian (dorsal spine).
The Gall Bladder Meridian (outer sides of torso).
Like all twists, this pose stimulates the liver and massages the stomach.

Anatomical Benefits

It helps release tension from the spine.
Placing the knees higher or lower will intensisfy the twist in the dorsal or lumbar spine respectively.

Contraindications

Shoulder issues.

Yang Sibling

Jathara Parivrtti (Revolved Abdomen Pose). In the Yang yoga version of this pose, we're actively aiding the twist instead of letting gravity do the work.

f you feel numbness or a tingling sensation in your raised arm or hand, use a variation of the pose!

MY NOTES

Mantra and Vibration:
A DIVINE PATH TO UNION

By David Lurey

Mantra, as part of Bhakti yoga, is a form of vibration through which we express our feelings and emotions. This vibration has a strong impact on those gathering together to chant and sing freely and can be a very liberating experience.

It is commonly accepted that the universe exists in vibration. From all matter in the material world to our emotions, thoughts and feelings, everything is vibrating. In yogic belief we can also assume that Divine Energy, the myriad forces that guide the universe into existence, are also vibrating. So we could say that through the sacred and powerful art of mantra chanting, we are harmonising our personal vibrations with that of the divine and entering the state of union/yoga with Divine Vibration.

As part of the path of Bhakti yoga, the yoga of devotion, chanting mantras is a selfless form of prayer that physiologically, emotionally and spiritually alters our vibrational state. Through singing, we vibrate the vocal chords and this resonates through the whole body. Muscles, bones, flesh and fluids all feel and receive the words. Through singing with intention, we bring our feelings out to the world and find new ways to express ourselves where others can feel them too.

One of the most common forms of chanting uses the different names of Hindu deities repeated over and over again to create a place of inner peace and union. This practice, called kirtan, takes advantage of the repetition to help calm the mind from constant distraction, which leads in turn to higher levels of presence. It is in the place where we are removed from our individual identity that we can feel more peace and be at one with God.

In many traditional schools, mantra chanting is a formal art to be practised under the guidance of a teacher to ensure proper pronunciation and recitation of the sacred words. Just as a specific recipe produces the same taste each time, traditional chanting utilises the internal vibrations of Sanskrit and the various names of gods and goddesses in a specific way as prescribed in ancient texts. These classical methods can be quite challenging for Westerners.

In many modern schools, however, the emphasis is on the intention behind the words and the calling out for union that makes an impact equal to that of the technique itself. With hundreds of thousands of people of many backgrounds discovering the joys of chanting, the vibrational effect of singing out loud is having a strong impact even if the exact pronunciation is missing. Many kirtan singers begin each chant with stories or basic translations for people to have some meaning behind the chants in their own language. When we can build these associations in our minds using words we know, the intention of each chant is set and has a greater potential to make an impact.

In yoga schools, ashrams, festivals and other gatherings around the world, modern kirtan singers are using Western instruments and melodies to create ecstatic kirtan and chanting and opening up brand-new feelings for practitioners. To sing freely and loudly without judgement and put a voice to the feelings inside is a very liberating act, and with music that supports the emotional release the experience can be very meditative (in both calming and exciting ways!).

As with most yogic practices, finding a balance between the more traditional fixed way and the modern artistic way can be found with mantra singing. Honouring the pronunciation and the sacredness of the words we sing while letting go of fear of doing the "wrong thing" can cultivate confidence in each of us to sing our own prayers. God will receive them gratefully!

My beloved kirtan teacher, Jai Uttal, says "there is no difference between God and the name of God". So each time we embark upon the journey of chanting, whether it is with classical monotonic melodies to cultivate an inner meditation or with modern upbeat music bringing an ecstatic joy, we are setting forth into the vibrational field with our own frequencies merging with the divine and ultimately bringing us to Yoga, Union.

"To sing freely and loudly without judgement and put a voice to the feelings inside is a very liberating act, and with music that supports the emotional release the experience can be very meditative."

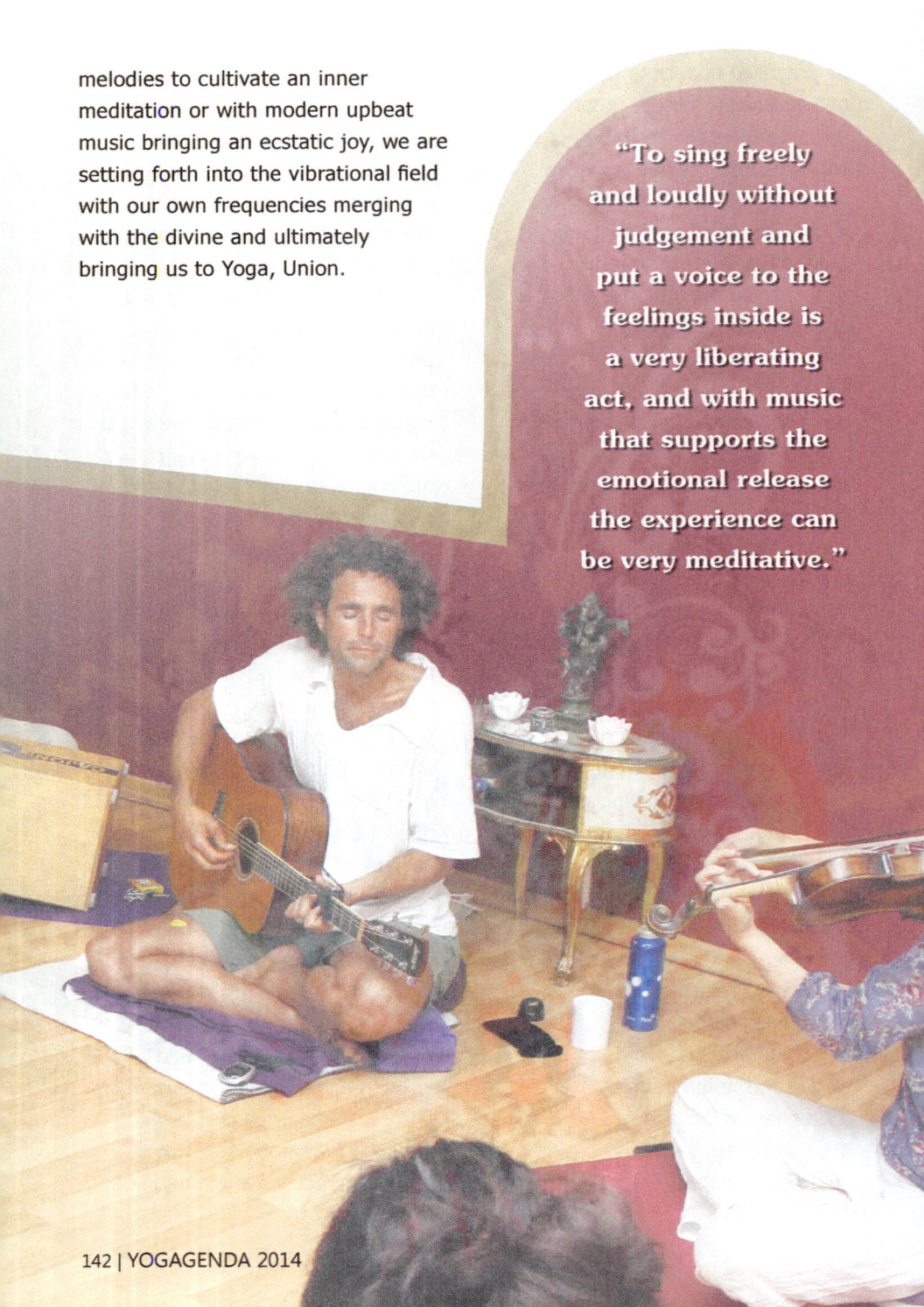

MY NOTES

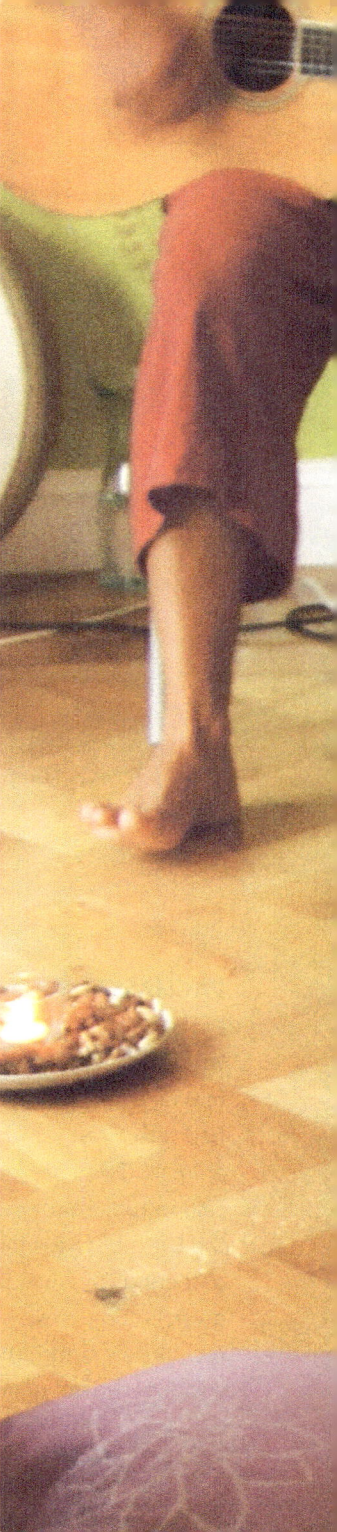

PACHAMAMA – Earth

Pachamama. It's a word most of us associate with the Earth and the feminine. But what does it really mean? The Pachamama is a representation of both the divine feminine and the physical Earth in Andean cultures. She is a mother figure concerned with fertility and generosity, and also a provider of protection for plants and animals. Often depicted as a huge dragon since she represents The Andes, she is said to cause earthquakes when disrespected. Pouring a few drops of a drink on the Earth before drinking is an act of reciprocity often performed during social gatherings by Andean people: the receiver says thank you and gives back to the giver. When we express gratitude for that received, somehow giving back to the receiver, we contribute to defuse the scarcity mindset so popular in our consumer societies; we are quenching the thirst of our souls with generosity of spirit.

August 2014

August 2014

					1	2	3
4	5	6	7	8	9	10	
11	12	13	14	15	16	17	
18	19	20	21	22	23	24	
25	26	27	28	29	30	31	

4
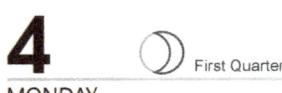 First Quarter

MONDAY

5
TUESDAY

6
WEDNESDAY

Sutra III.31 *kantha kupe ksut pipasa nivrttih*

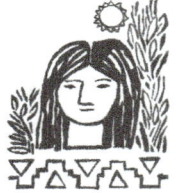

7
THURSDAY

8
FRIDAY

9
SATURDAY

Full Moon ◯

Super Full Moon

10
SUNDAY

August 2014

				1	2	3
4	5	6	7	8	9	10
11	12	13	14	15	16	17
18	19	20	21	22	23	24
25	26	27	28	29	30	31

week 32

August 2014

11
MONDAY

12
TUESDAY

13
WEDNESDAY

Sutra III.32 *kurmanadyam sthairyam*

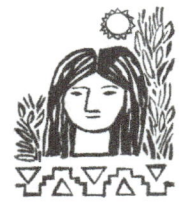

14
THURSDAY

15
FRIDAY

16
SATURDAY

Last Quarter 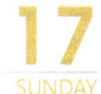 # 17
SUNDAY

August 2014

				1	2	3
4	5	6	7	8	9	10
11	12	13	14	15	16	17
18	19	20	21	22	23	24
25	26	27	28	29	30	31

week 33

August 2014

18
MONDAY

19
TUESDAY

20
WEDNESDAY

Sutra III.33 *murdha jyotisi siddha darsanam*

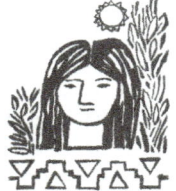

21
THURSDAY

22
FRIDAY

23
SATURDAY

24
SUNDAY

August 2014

				1	2	3
4	5	6	7	8	9	10
11	12	13	14	15	16	17
18	19	20	21	22	23	24
25	26	27	28	29	30	31

week 34

August 2014

25
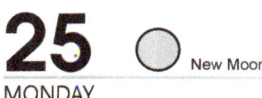 New Moon
MONDAY

26
TUESDAY

27
WEDNESDAY

Sutra III.34 *pratibhad va sarvam*

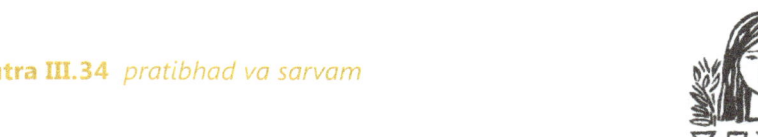

28
THURSDAY

29
FRIDAY

30
SATURDAY

31
SUNDAY

August 2014

					1	2	3
4	5	6	7	8	9	10
11	12	13	14	15	16	17
18	19	20	21	22	23	24
25	26	27	28	29	30	31

week 35

SPHINX
Spleen Meridian

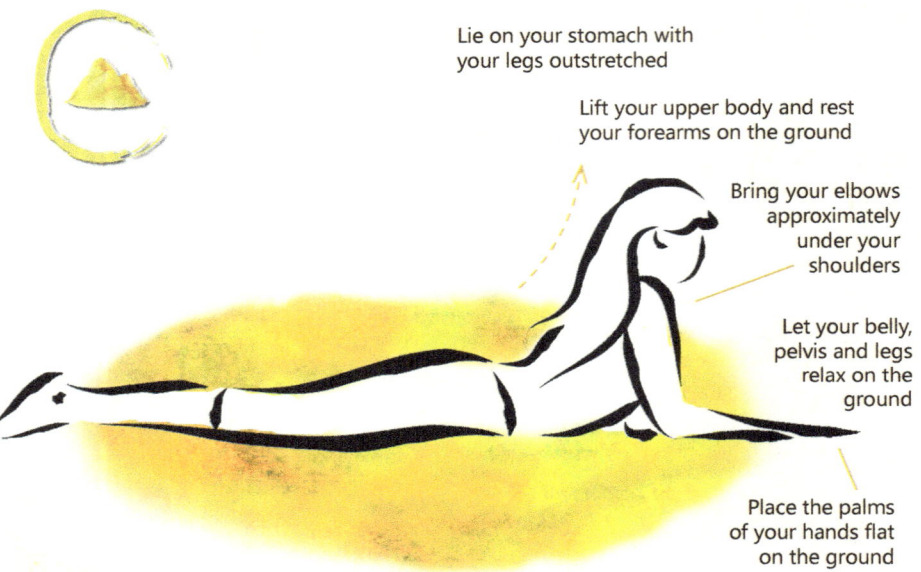

Lie on your stomach with your legs outstretched

Lift your upper body and rest your forearms on the ground

Bring your elbows approximately under your shoulders

Let your belly, pelvis and legs relax on the ground

Place the palms of your hands flat on the ground

While in the Pose

- Holding time: 1 to 5 minutes.
- Breathe deeply and mindfully.

Coming out of the Pose

- Leave the pose slowly and mindfully.
- Exhale, move your elbows out to the sides and come down to lie on your stomach, resting your head on your hands.
- Whenever you feel ready, press yourself gently back into Balasana (Child's Pose) on an exhalation. Move your knees approximately mat-distance apart, so that you can rest your torso in between your legs.
- Observe the effects of the pose.

Modifications and Variations

- If you feel a painful compression in your lumbar spine, bring your elbows further forwards so your ribs rest more fully on the ground.
- Place your head on a block or cushion if your neck feels too tense.

Taking it Further

- Place a cushion under your elbows to further lift your chest.
- Bend your knees or spread your legs apart for further sacral compression.
- Come into Seal Pose: extend your arms fully with your palms flat on the ground; your hands can be turned outwards, inwards, facing forwards or towards your body.

Meridians and Organs Affected

The Spleen and Stomach meridians (front of torso).
The Kidney and Urinary Bladder meridians (lumbar and sacral area).
It stimulates the kidneys and suprarenal glands when compressing the lower back.

Anatomical Benefits

It creates healthy stress on the lumbar and sacral area, helping to regenerate the lower lumbar spinal curve.
It tones the entire spine.

Contraindications

Avoid if the sacral area is very tight or injured.
Pressing the belly into the ground during pregnancy is not recommended.

Yang Sibling

Salamba Bhujangasana (Sphinx Pose). In the Yang yoga version of this pose, we take the tailbone towards the pubic bone to lengthen the lower back. The legs are active and the upper torso is actively lifting up.

If you feel any painful sensation in your neck or sacrum, use a variation of the pose!

MY NOTES

Durga:
THE GODDESS OF
A THOUSAND FACES

By Irantzu Piquero

One of the many stories of Mother Earth, this time in her incarnation as Durga, reminding us of our potential as warriors and bringers of harmony despite our tendency to become mired in negative life patterns.

There was a time when the Earth was worshipped as Mother Goddess, an infinite source of creativity, protection, nourishment and shelter. In India it had a thousand names. One of them is Sri Lakshmi, the Lotus Goddess, who extends her arms in a gesture of generosity so we can resonate with her vast abundance: that quality of the universe to endlessly create.

At some point in time, she was silenced. A whole pantheon of armed warrior gods tried to reflect the different aspects of Mother Nature. The earthly, the physical, became an obstacle that needed to be transcended. Spirituality turned towards the celestial, the pure, towards liberation. The goddess was muted and she was called a Mirage, Poison, an Illusion. But a few centuries of silence is only a blink of the eye for her as she watches mountains and continents come and go, like we watch the waves ebb and flow...

There's an ancient story in the sacred Hindu text Devi Mahatmya, within the Markandeya Puranas, about the return of the goddess after hundreds or thousands of years away. It tells how a buffalo-demon called Mahisa terrorised the world. The devas or gods went to Brahma for help and he in turn called Vishnu and Shiva, who, furious, released a flare of fire from their eyes and mouths. The gods joined them, shooting out burning flames. And from the fire, the devi or goddess Durga materialised. In this way, all that was taken away was returned to her. The vital energy, the shakti, of each one of the gods returned to its source: to the spring from where everything stems, the Mother.

Each of the devas presented Durga a gift: Shiva his trident; Vishnu his whirling fiery discus; Indra his thunderbolt; Kubera offered a cup; the god's architect Vishvakarman, and the eternal serpent Ananta, honoured her with adornments; and the god of the Himalayas gave her his mount, a lion. With a fierce smile, Durga raised up her eight arms filling the cosmos with light. Beautiful and dangerous, she let out a roar that made the universe tremble.

Mahisa heard the call and set out to confront her. His never-ending army of asuras initiated the combat, and Durga and her lion charged like a flame in a dry forest, submerging the demons in an ocean of blood.

Durga is the capacity to fight in each woman, our warrioress-like potential. It makes us strong and resolute when a cycle finishes, blessing the Earth with blood to let a new cycle begin afresh. After defeating the demon's vassals, the Goddess prepared herself to receive him. And Mahisa, breaking the earth with his hooves, throwing mountains at her as he advanced, charged to make his offering...

The devi threw Mahisa a rope and he turned it into a lion whose head Durga cut off. The lion then became a giant warrior armed with a scimitar, but she took him down with her arrows. He then transformed into an elephant who knocked down Durga's mount with his trunk, then recovered his buffalo shape. The goddess stood up and the three worlds held their breath.

Are you able to see when a situation repeats itself? When a problem recurs again and again, only under a different guise?

Durga laughed. She saluted Mahisa with her cup filled with amrita, the nectar of the gods, and after emptying it, she threw herself into a final attack until the buffalo bit the dust under her feet. And Durga, calm and graceful, raised her trophy at last.

Durga continues to be the Great Mother, the primary cosmic force, the origin of everything. With her return and her battle, she restores harmony and placates the destructive and entwined forces that deplete the Earth's resources in an orgy of self-indulgent irresponsibility. She invites us to passionately embrace our own inner fire: our life.

Durga is the warrioress and bloody goddess. There will be other manifestations of the goddess, other times that will call for a return of her sweeter aspects. But that's a different story to be told on a different occasion...

> **"Durga is the capacity to fight in each woman, our warrioress-like potential. It makes us strong and resolute when a cycle finishes, blessing the Earth with blood to let a new cycle begin afresh."**

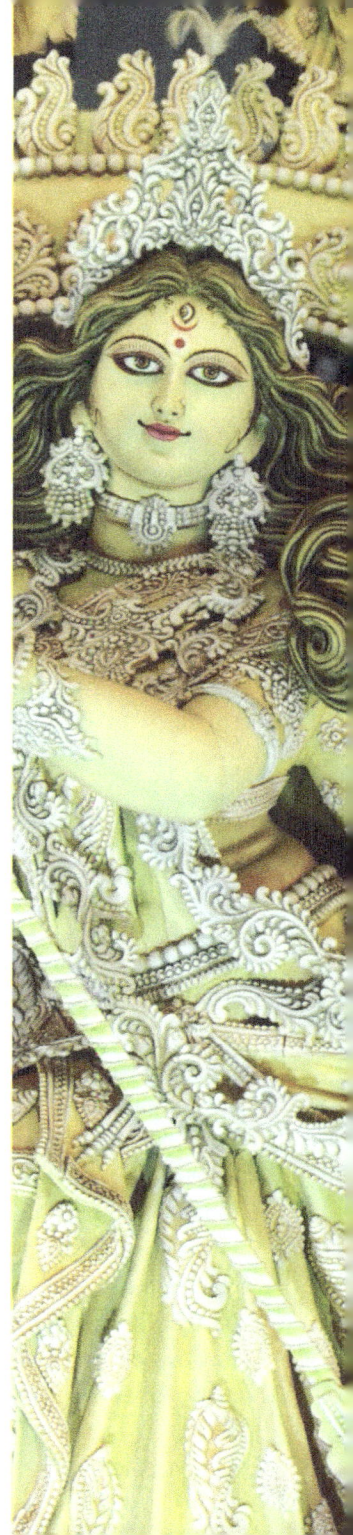

MOUNTAINS – Earth

Despite occupying a quarter of the land's surface, mountain areas are sparsely populated. Life conditions are more favourable, for example, in valleys or next to the sea than at high altitudes. It is perhaps for this reason that mountains are symbolic of obstacles to conquer. And if a high peak is the closest we can get to Heaven from Earth, the conquering effort is not devoid of reward! Traditionally, mountains also stand for constancy, stillness or firmness, values that point towards a certain quality of effort. So mountains are symbolic both of a challenge and the response to a challenge – or wise effort. Cosmic mountains in some traditions have a world axis or centre that connects Heaven and Earth. In yoga, our body is that axis or centre, and as we practise sincerely to align ourselves with our true being, creative response to challenge naturally develops in us.

September 2014

September 2014

1	2	3	4	5	6	7
8	9	10	11	12	13	14
15	16	17	18	19	20	21
22	23	24	25	26	27	28
29	30					

September 2014

1
MONDAY

2
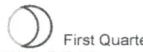 First Quarter

TUESDAY

3
WEDNESDAY

Sutra III.35 *hrdaye citta samvit*

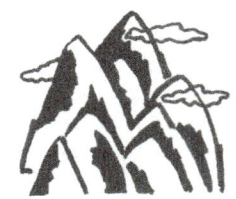

4
THURSDAY

5
FRIDAY

6
SATURDAY

7
SUNDAY

September 2014

1	2	3	4	5	6	7	week 36
8	9	10	11	12	13	14	
15	16	17	18	19	20	21	
22	23	24	25	26	27	28	
29	30						

September 2014

8
MONDAY

9
TUESDAY

○ Full Moon

10
WEDNESDAY

Sutra III.36 *sattva purusayor atyantasamkirnayoh
pratyayaviseso bhogah pararthat
svarthasamyamat purusa jnanam*

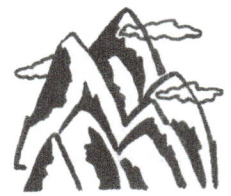

11
THURSDAY

12
FRIDAY

13
SATURDAY

14
SUNDAY

September 2014

1	2	3	4	5	6	7
8	9	10	11	12	13	14
15	16	17	18	19	20	21
22	23	24	25	26	27	28
29	30					

week 37

September 2014

15
MONDAY

16 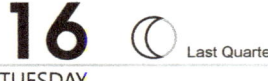 Last Quarter
TUESDAY

17
WEDNESDAY

Sutra III.37 *tatah pratibha sravana vedanadarsasvada varta jayante*

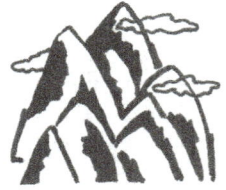

18
THURSDAY

19
FRIDAY

20
SATURDAY

21
SUNDAY

September 2014

1	2	3	4	5	6	7	
8	9	10	11	12	13	14	
15	16	17	18	19	20	21	week 38
22	23	24	25	26	27	28	
29	30						

22
MONDAY

23
TUESDAY   Autumn Equinox

24
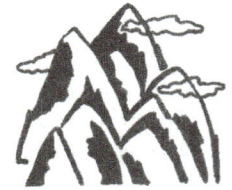 New Moon
WEDNESDAY

Sutra III.38 *te samadhav upasarga vyutthane siddhayh*

25
THURSDAY

26
FRIDAY

27
SATURDAY

28
SUNDAY

September 2014

1	2	3	4	5	6	7
8	9	10	11	12	13	14
15	16	17	18	19	20	21
22	23	24	25	26	27	28
29	30					

week 39

DRAGON FLYING HIGH
Stomach Meridian

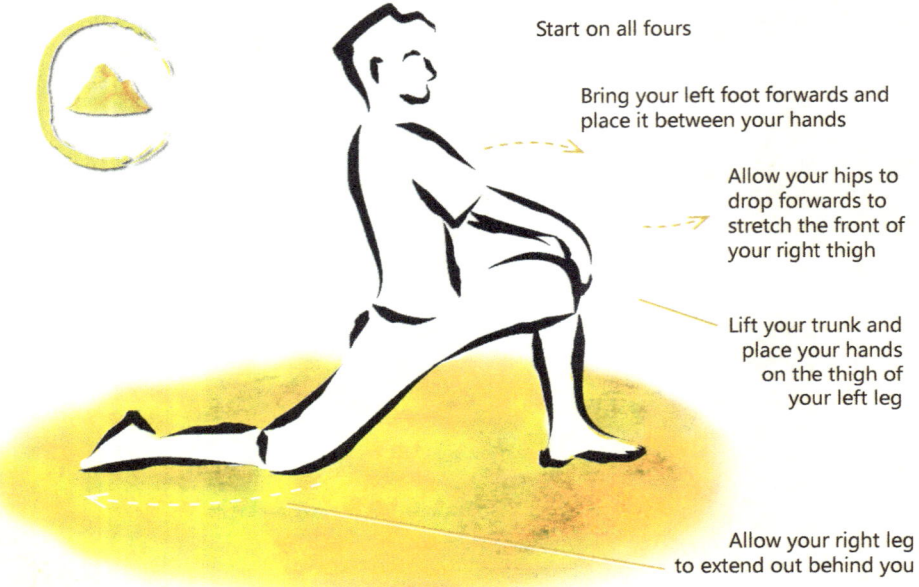

Start on all fours

Bring your left foot forwards and place it between your hands

Allow your hips to drop forwards to stretch the front of your right thigh

Lift your trunk and place your hands on the thigh of your left leg

Allow your right leg to extend out behind you

While in the Pose

- Holding time: 1 to 5 minutes on each side.
- Breathe deeply and mindfully.

Coming out of the Pose

- Leave the pose slowly and mindfully.
- Slowly and gently take your front leg back for a short Adho Mukha Svanasana (Downward-Facing Dog). Bend your knees, stretching one leg out at a time. On an exhalation, relax down to Balasana (Child's Pose).
- Observe the effects of the pose.

Modifications and Variations

- Use a blanket to protect your knee or ankle if necessary.
- Rest your elbows on your front knee, or your hands on the ground or on blocks, and bring your trunk lower if you feel a painful compression in the lower back.

Taking it Further

- Wing out your front leg to get deeper into this hip.
- From the initial position, bring both hands to the inside of the front leg and walk them forwards to further stretch your hips. You can also place your forearms on the ground to intensify the stretch.

Meridians and Organs Affected

The Stomach, Spleen and Kidney meridians (front of torso and front and inner legs).
The Liver meridian (inner legs).
The Urinary Bladder meridian (back of legs and lumbar spine).
The kidneys receive a gentle massage if there is healthy stress on the lumbar area.

Anatomical Benefits

It deeply opens the hips and groins.
It stretches the back leg's hip flexors and frontal thigh.
It also stretches the front leg's back thigh.

Contraindications

Knee problems.

Yang Sibling

Anjaneyasana (Low Lunge). In the Yang yoga version of this pose, the front knee is directly above the front ankle. The tailbone is drawing down towards the ground and the pubic bone towards the navel to stretch the spine.

If you feel any painful sensation in your knee or ankle, use a variation of the pose!

MY NOTES

Fascia:
THE GLUE THAT HOLDS OUR BODY TOGETHER

By Mirjam Wagner

There is a tissue in the human body that is often neglected in many anatomy books although it is one of the most important: the fascia. It's time to consciously include it in our practice through appropriate Yin or Yang poses and to enjoy the amazing results.

We are all made of fascia. Every single one of our muscles and nerve fibres are wrapped in a thin membrane of fascia. Groups of fibres are also held together by other fascious membranes and the same type of tissue connects the muscles and organs to the bones and interconnects them with each other.

The fascia has three very different functions to perform:
- to give stability and hold the different tissues together.
- to provide elasticity and give each bone and organ enough space for their movements and functions.
- to transport prana through the energy channels of the body.

Seeing how different these functions are, even though it is the same tissue, it is important that we have a better understanding of it, as well as how we can enhance each of the independent functions without neglecting another through the practice of Yin or Yang yoga (see pp.106-108).

Fascia is made of water, collagen and elastane.

- Water serves as the base in which the energy channels are conducting prana throughout the body. If there are any blockages in the fascia, energy gets stuck and our health is in danger.
- Collagen fibres act like glue, providing stability at joints and other places where different structures need to connect with each other.
- Elastane fibres bring elasticity into the fascia, so that a certain amount of movement is guaranteed.

For example, let's look at the hip joint. This ball-and-socket type of joint allows a wide range of movement, while also giving tremendous stability to walk through life with strong legs, plus having the responsibility of dealing with the weight of the whole upper body.

How can we increase stability without losing elasticity in the hip joint?

"I am often asked in my workshops and anatomy classes: "Isn't it dangerous to stretch ligaments and tendons?" We must allow ligaments, tendons and other fascia the opportunity to let go, receive positive stress and become more elastic and stronger. But we need to know how to reach these tissues without risking injury."

The ligaments, tendons and joint capsule of the hip joint (each one of them a type of fascia or connective tissue) hold the head of the femur bone attached to the acetabulum (the cavity within the pelvic bones)

and provides stability at this joint. To enhance this function we must ensure conscious muscle action and proper alignment in standing Yang poses.

How can we become more flexible in the hip joint without losing stability and strength?

The elastane particles in the ligaments and tendons have the capacity to let go in an appropriate way and allow the femur bone to move in different directions. Holding a Yin pose for several minutes (e.g., Butterfly Pose, see pp.104-105) with relaxed muscles helps the fascia in this target area to gain more elasticity and opens the hip joint on a very deep level; this way we provide a wider range of movement at this joint and obtain more flexibility.

I am often asked in my workshops and anatomy classes: "Isn't it dangerous to stretch ligaments and tendons?" We must allow ligaments, tendons and other fascia the opportunity to let go, receive positive stress and become more elastic and stronger. But we need to know how to reach these tissues without risking injury.

The fascia itself can not contract voluntarily, however over time it tightens and loses elasticity with age and immobility. Fascia needs time to let go and stay healthy and elastic. Yin yoga is an excellent tool to reach these tissues without injury. If we want the fascia around a joint to take full advantage in a Yin pose, the muscles of the target area must be completely relaxed. Relaxed muscles create more space between the bones adding positive stress to the tendons and ligaments and balancing strength and flexibility in the fascia.

Every ligament has a different structure and composition of collagen and elastane depending on their location and function. So ligaments whose function is more about stability, like the cruciate ligaments of the knee, need less mobility and therefore less "stretching" than ligaments whose function is more for mobility, like those around the spine.

Let's give the fascia in our body more attention! Treat them to appropriate poses with time to let go and you will be rewarded with strength and flexibility that allows healthy organs, deep breathing and unblocked emotions.

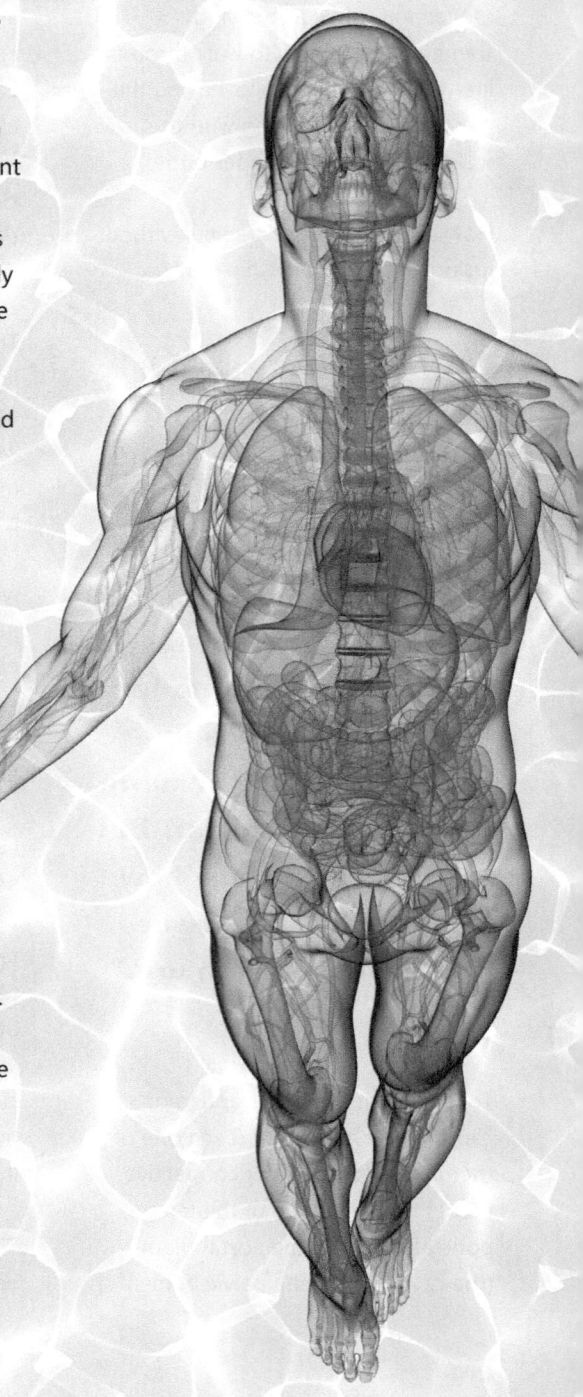

VAJRA – Metal

In the Buddhist tradition, a vajra is a ritual object that symbolises simultaneously the qualities of a diamond and a thunderbolt. Diamonds are hard, and cutting or scratching them is very difficult. A thunderbolt, on the other hand, is a force able to shatter almost everything it comes into contact with. In a vajra, the diamond stands for indestructibility and the thunderbolt for irresistible force. It is a symbol of spiritual power: that which is enduring and invincible. In Hatha yoga, there is a pose called Vajrasana or Thunderbolt pose, in which we kneel with our knees together and sit on our calves (with a folded blanket beneath our sitting bones if necessary). In this asana, the spine is alert allowing the flow of energy along it. If we spend time in it cultivating meditative awareness, we will open the doors of our own spiritual power.

October 2014

JOURNAL

October 2014

		1	2	3	4	5
6	7	8	9	10	11	12
13	14	15	16	17	18	19
20	21	22	23	24	25	26
27	28	29	30	31		

29
MONDAY

30
TUESDAY

1
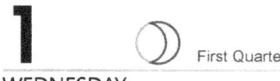 First Quarter

WEDNESDAY

Sutra III.39 *bandha karana saithilyat pracara samvedanac ca cittasya parasariravesah*

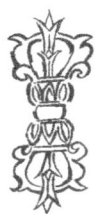

2
THURSDAY

3
FRIDAY

4
SATURDAY

5
SUNDAY

October 2014

		1	2	3	4	5	week 40
6	7	8	9	10	11	12	
13	14	15	16	17	18	19	
20	21	22	23	24	25	26	
27	28	29	30	31			

6
MONDAY

7
TUESDAY

8 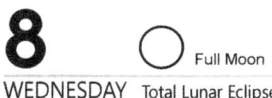 Full Moon
WEDNESDAY Total Lunar Eclipse

Sutra III.40 *udana jayaj jala panka kantakadisv asanga utkrantis ca*

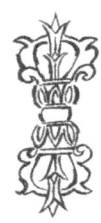

9
THURSDAY

10
FRIDAY

11
SATURDAY

12
SUNDAY

October 2014

	1	2	3	4	5	
6	7	8	9	10	11	12
13	14	15	16	17	18	19
20	21	22	23	24	25	26
27	28	29	30	31		

week 41

13
MONDAY

14
TUESDAY

15 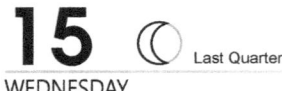 Last Quarter
WEDNESDAY

Sutra III.41 *samana jayaj jvalanam*

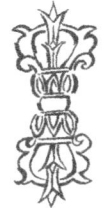

16
THURSDAY

17
FRIDAY

18
SATURDAY

19
SUNDAY

October 2014

		1	2	3	4	5
6	7	8	9	10	11	12
13	14	15	16	17	18	19
20	21	22	23	24	25	26
27	28	29	30	31		

week 42

October 2014

20
MONDAY

21
TUESDAY

22
WEDNESDAY

Sutra III.42 *srotrakasayoh sambandha samyamad divyam*
srotram

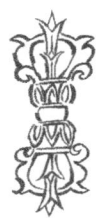

New Moon ◯ **23**
Partial Solar Eclipse   **THURSDAY**

24
FRIDAY

25
SATURDAY

26
SUNDAY

October 2014

		1	2	3	4	5
6	7	8	9	10	11	12
13	14	15	16	17	18	19
20	21	22	23	24	25	26
27	28	29	30	31		

week 43

October 2014

27
MONDAY

28
TUESDAY

29
WEDNESDAY

Sutra III.43 *kayakasayoh sambandha samyamal laghu tula*
samapattes cakasa gamanam

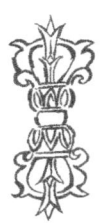

30
THURSDAY

First Quarter ◗ # 31
FRIDAY

1
SATURDAY

2
SUNDAY

October 2014

		1	2	3	4	5
6	7	8	9	10	11	12
13	14	15	16	17	18	19
20	21	22	23	24	25	26
27	28	29	30	31		

week 44

BANANASANA WITH ARMS UP
Lung Meridian

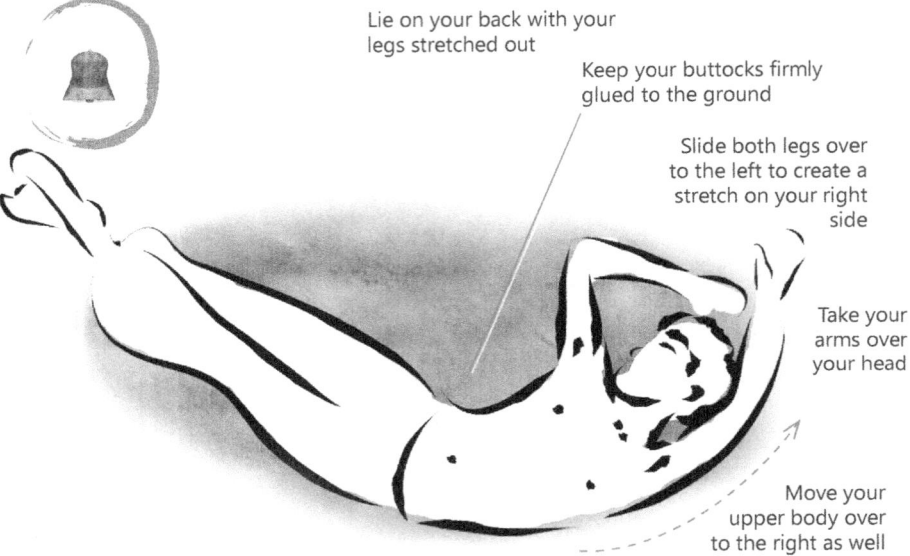

Lie on your back with your legs stretched out

Keep your buttocks firmly glued to the ground

Slide both legs over to the left to create a stretch on your right side

Take your arms over your head

Move your upper body over to the right as well

While in the Pose

- Holding time: 3 to 15 minutes on each side.
- Breathe deeply and mindfully.

Coming out of the Pose

- Leave the pose slowly and mindfully.
- Come back to a neutral position before doing the other side.
- Exhale and bring your arms down. Extend your legs first and then bring your knees to your chest.
- Hug your lower legs and circle your knees to massage the lumbar and sacral area.
- Observe the effects of the pose.

Modifications and Variations

- Rest your arms over your chest if you feel numbness in your arms or hands.
- You can choose a different pose with arms outstretched to affect the Lung meridian, such as Butterfly (see pp.104-105) with the palm of your hands together and arms stretched on the floor in front of you.

Taking it Further

- Interlace your fingers or take hold of opposite elbows.
- Play with crossing your outer ankle over your inner ankle and the other way around.

Meridians and Organs Affected

The Lung and Heart meridians (outer and inner arms).
The Gall Bladder meridian (outer sides of torso).
It stimulates the stomach, liver and intestines.

Anatomical Benefits

It deeply stretches one side of the body while creating healthy stress on the other.
It also stretches the outer hips and outer legs.

Contraindications

Shoulder issues.
Serious lumbar injuries.

Yang Sibling

The Half Moon version included at the beginning of Chandra Namaskara (Moon Salutation) is a similar side bend pose, although standing.

If you feel any numbness or tingling sensation in your arms, use a variation of the pose!

MY NOTES

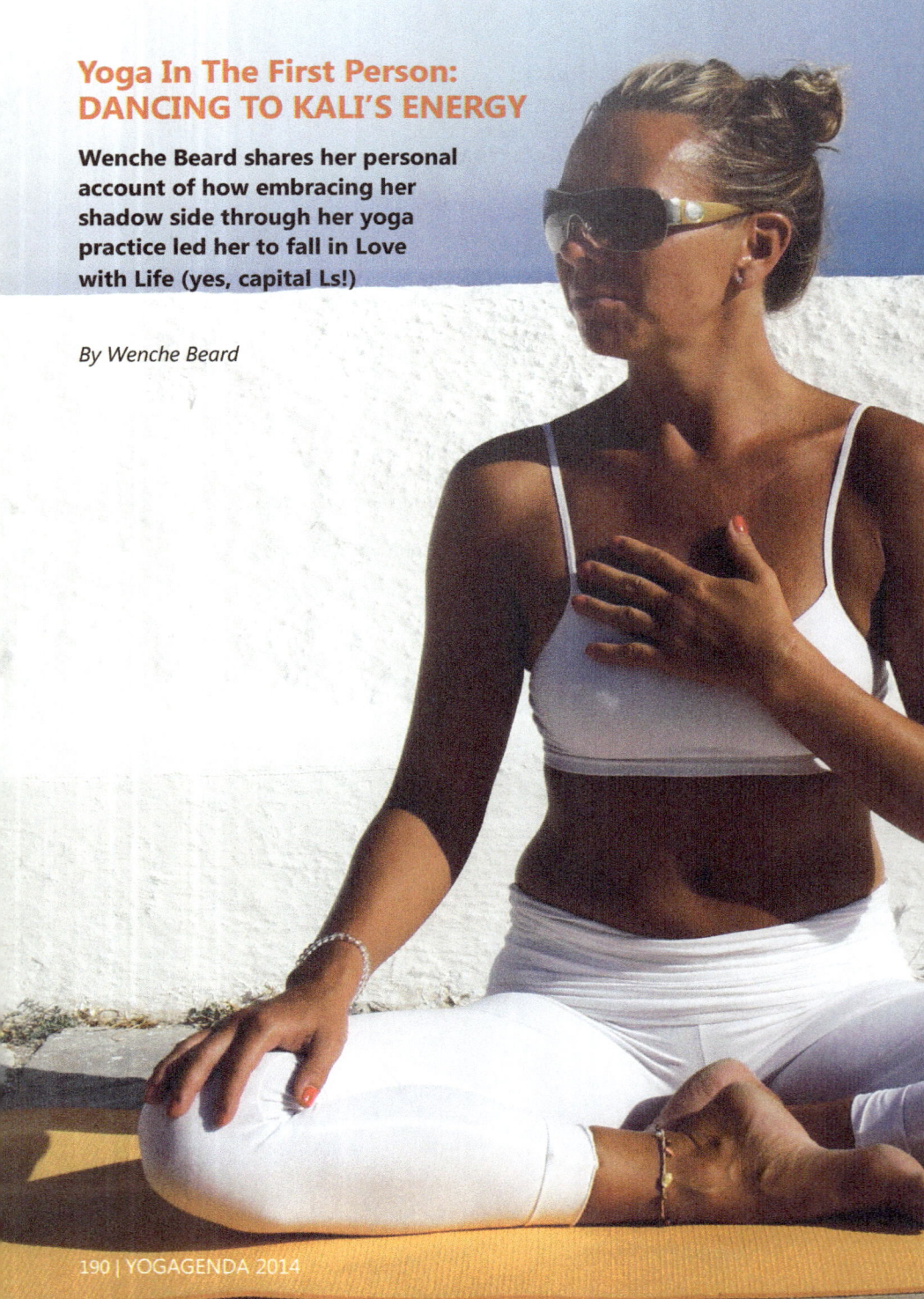

Yoga In The First Person:
DANCING TO KALI'S ENERGY

Wenche Beard shares her personal account of how embracing her shadow side through her yoga practice led her to fall in Love with Life (yes, capital Ls!)

By Wenche Beard

It is my experience that there is a yoga practice for everyone, no matter what your physical, mental or emotional state. Yoga is clever: it brings light and hope into our darkest corners; it transforms our shadows into light...

It was during my yoga teacher training that my teacher first explained to me about my shadow side. It was important too and why did I keep avoiding it? What did he mean? Of course I wanted to avoid it, who wouldn't? My teacher suggested it was time to meet it. He explained that we could do this by working with the energy of Kali. Kali is the Hindu goddess of endings and beginnings. Her energy helps to battle your demons and cut through delusions. From a yogic aspect Kali holds a dark and transcendent energy of real power and presence. She teaches us that we all have this interplay with light and shadow in our lives and allows us to transform from darkness to light.

My shadow appeared to me as a face I could not see clearly. I became aware that the face I was frightened of seeing was me. My fears prevented me from dancing my dance. I realised I had to reclaim the parts of me I had given to fear; fear was not serving me. I became curious and began to explore my practice. I dived into the liberating qualities of apas (water) that nourishes our joy and inherent freedom to move and feel. I incorporated a powerful agni (fire) practice serving the absorption and purifying process within body and mind. I "danced" with Kali, the dance of destruction, the dance of change.

As I began to explore the Kali energy I grew even stronger, I met myself and others with greater confidence and power. I learned the art of letting go, I learned to love me. By embracing my shadow with compassion and understanding, my heart grew and the colours of the rainbow became even brighter. I felt a love for life beyond my wildest dreams. Through Kali's strength I am moving out of fear into following my heart's true desires. When we find the courage to follow our wildest dreams,

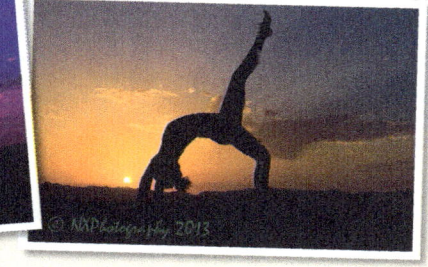

we make changes not just within ourselves, but in our life, in our community and in the world.

My journey has been a beautiful experience, and for the last 13 years it has taken me on a quest to share yoga with beings everywhere. Yoga has become the foundation of strength for all my clients whatever background, religion or health issue. It has given hope to my mental health students. It brings them light and hope in an often dark and scary world. The energy at the closed unit where I teach is often stagnant, dark and heavy; and this is their home. I see how yoga brightens their day. Their commitment is incredible and the benefits many. My reward is when they smile, and for a split second light comes into their eyes. I watch them surrendering into the present and their world

becoming brighter and lighter, giving them hope.

This is a real contrast to the settings and the personal environment of yoga enthusiasts on my yoga holidays. Here we may practice yoga on a beautiful beach while listening to the sound of the waves lapping on the shore. The situation and the people couldn't be more different, but in some ways we are all the same. You see we all breathe, move and heal. We are all longing for that same thing: to become who we really are, free from fear, to feel unconditional Love and Joy. That is our birth right. We all just want to be healthy and happy.

Yoga is like starting a love affair with ourselves. It allows us to connect with our creative power, our passion and the ability to feel – and when we really feel, we heal. Yoga fills us with inner richness, like a smile rising from the depths of silence and spreading through the breath of grace.

TRISHULA – Metal

This three-pointed weapon is an attribute often present in the iconography of numerous deities. Shiva wields a Trishula; he is the Hindu god of destruction, following Vishnu the preserver, who himself follows Brahma the creator in an endless cycle of change. As a weapon of Shiva, the trishula is said to destroy the physical world, the world of our ancestors (culture drawn from the past), and the world of the mind (the ego and any false identification with the form, including useless habits and attachments). Shiva stands for letting go of everything in the world of form and his power of destruction has a purifying effect; it ends the illusion of permanence and individuality so a blissful non-dual plane of existence can emerge. His message is clear: regeneration is inherent to destruction and there are seeds of new opportunities in every loss.

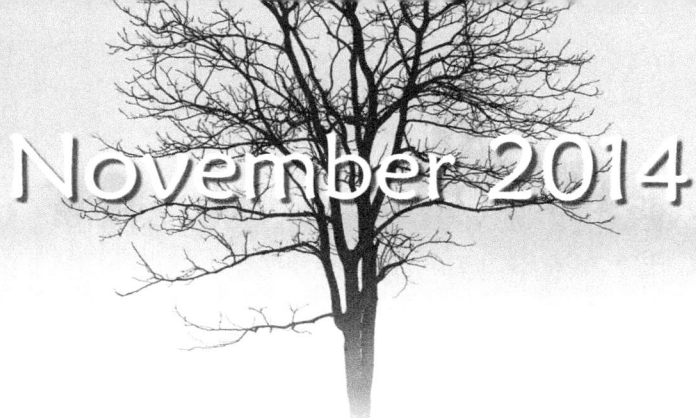

November 2014

November 2014

					1	2
3	4	5	6	7	8	9
10	11	12	13	14	15	16
17	18	19	20	21	22	23
24	25	26	27	28	29	30

November 2014

3
MONDAY

4
TUESDAY

5
WEDNESDAY

Sutra III.44 *bahir akalpita vrttir mahavideha tatah*
prakasavarana ksayah

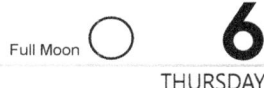

Full Moon

6
THURSDAY

7
FRIDAY

8
SATURDAY

9
SUNDAY

November 2014

					1	2
3	4	5	6	7	8	9
10	11	12	13	14	15	16
17	18	19	20	21	22	23
24	25	26	27	28	29	30

week 45

10
MONDAY

11
TUESDAY

12
WEDNESDAY

Sutra III.45 *sthula svarupa suksmanvayarthavattva
samyamad bhutajayah*

13
THURSDAY

Last Quarter **14**
FRIDAY

15
SATURDAY

16
SUNDAY

November 2014

					1	2
3	4	5	6	7	8	9
10	11	12	13	14	15	16
17	18	19	20	21	22	23
24	25	26	27	28	29	30

week 46

17
MONDAY

18
TUESDAY

19
WEDNESDAY

Sutra III.46 *tatonimadi pradurbhavah kaya sampat taddharmanabhighatas ca*

20
THURSDAY

21
FRIDAY

New Moon ⃝ **22**
SATURDAY

23
SUNDAY

November 2014

					1	2
3	4	5	6	7	8	9
10	11	12	13	14	15	16
17	18	19	20	21	22	23
24	25	26	27	28	29	30

week 47

24
MONDAY

25
TUESDAY

26
WEDNESDAY

Sutra III.47 *rupa lavanya bala vajrasamhananatvani kayasampat*

27
THURSDAY

28
FRIDAY

First Quarter 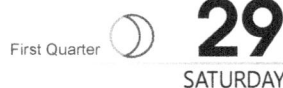 ## 29
SATURDAY

30
SUNDAY

November 2014

					1	2
3	4	5	6	7	8	9
10	11	12	13	14	15	16
17	18	19	20	21	22	23
24	25	26	27	28	29	30

week 48

DRAGONFLY TWIST
Large Intestine Meridian

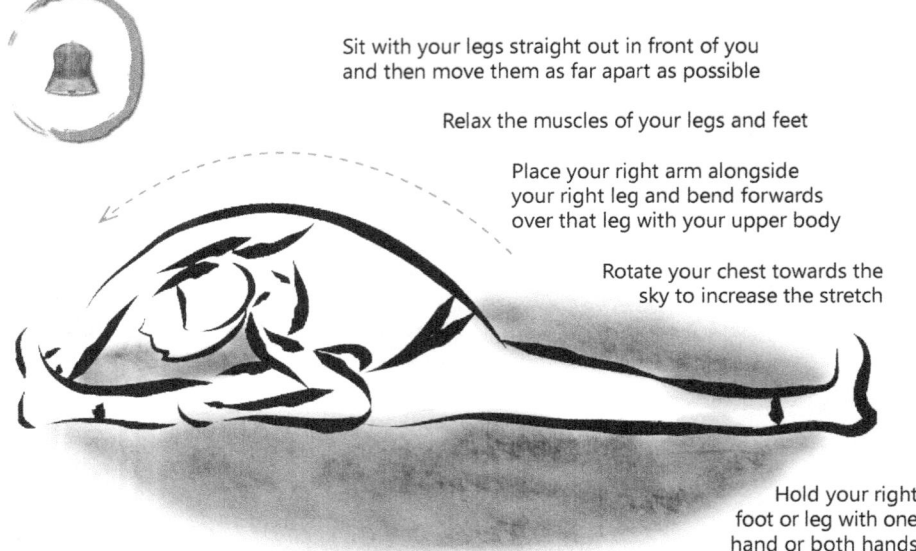

Sit with your legs straight out in front of you and then move them as far apart as possible

Relax the muscles of your legs and feet

Place your right arm alongside your right leg and bend forwards over that leg with your upper body

Rotate your chest towards the sky to increase the stretch

Hold your right foot or leg with one hand or both hands

While in the Pose

- Holding time: 3 to 5 minutes on each side.
- Breathe deeply and mindfully.

Coming out of the Pose

- Leave the pose slowly and mindfully.
- Inhale and slowly raise your body back up to the centre. Bend your legs with the help of your hands and place your feet flat on the ground in front of you.
- Bring your knees together and embrace your lower legs, resting your forehead on your knees.
- Observe the effects of the pose.

Modifications and Variations

- If you have any knee issues, bring your legs closer together and/or slightly bend your knees.
- Place a blanket under your knees if the back of your thighs feel tight.
- Sit on a folded blanket to elevate your hips if your lower back hurts or you suffer from sciatica.
- Rest your head on your hand if it feels too heavy.

Taking it Further

- Hold the back of your right thigh with your left hand (when folding towards the right) and then repeat on the other side.

Meridians and Organs Affected

The Large Intestine meridian (outer arms).
The Kidney and Liver meridians (groins and inner legs).
The Spleen meridian (inner knees).
The Gall Bladder meridian (outer sides of torso).
It massages the ovaries and stimulates the liver.

Anatomical Benefits

It stretches the groins, and the back and inner sides of the thighs.
It opens up the inner knees.
It elongates the outer sides of the torso.
It creates healthy stress on the hips.

Contraindications

Inner knee issues.
Lower back injuries.

Yang Sibling

Upavistha Konasana Twist (Wide-Angle Seated Forward Bend with Twist).
In the Yang yoga version of this pose, the legs are active and the feet are in flex and the lower side of the body kept as long as possible.

If you feel any painful sensation in your knees or lower back, use a variation of the pose!

MY NOTES

To Eat Or Not To Eat:
A YOGIC DIET

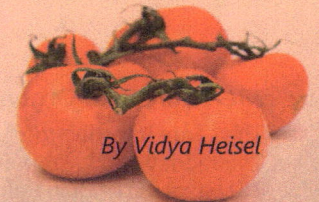

By Vidya Heisel

Yoga has always embraced a very holistic approach to health and many guidelines about personal hygiene and diet can be found in the ancient yogic texts. But how does traditional dietary advice relate to our present-day lives?

In yogic philosophy the manifest world (prakriti) is made up of three types of energies or gunas: sattva, rajas and tamas. In everything that exists, one of these forms of energy is predominant, although it may also contain elements of the other two.

Sattva is the purest form of energy. Its characteristics are light, pure, clear and peaceful. Rajas is the energy of movement, change, action, passion and restlessness. Tamas is the more sluggish energy of ego, laziness and inertia (think couch potato and junk food). Everything in existence dances between these three states and they are all necessary. A human being can be in a sattvic state when meditating, rajasic when going for a run and tamasic when asleep.

Food, being manifest matter, falls into all three of these energy categories. What we eat not only affects how we look physically, but also how we feel and how clear and creative our mental energy is. Some foods support and enliven our yoga practice and life-force energy, whilst other foods inhibit and undermine them. If the food we are eating contains sattvic energy, the body simply becomes more sattvic by eating it. One of the goals of yogis is to become more sattvic, therefore eating predominantly sattvic foods is considered the best yogic diet.

A sattvic diet supports good health as well as, importantly, the practice of meditation and yoga asana. All fresh fruit, vegetables, nuts, seeds, legumes and whole-grains are considered sattvic. Dairy is also deemed sattvic. However, we should bear in mind that the dairy that ancient yogis ate was probably limited amounts of raw buffalo milk, simple plain home-made yogurt and paneer, the most basic form of cheese made by curdling milk with lemon juice. This form of dairy was not pasteurised, homogenised, or made with any

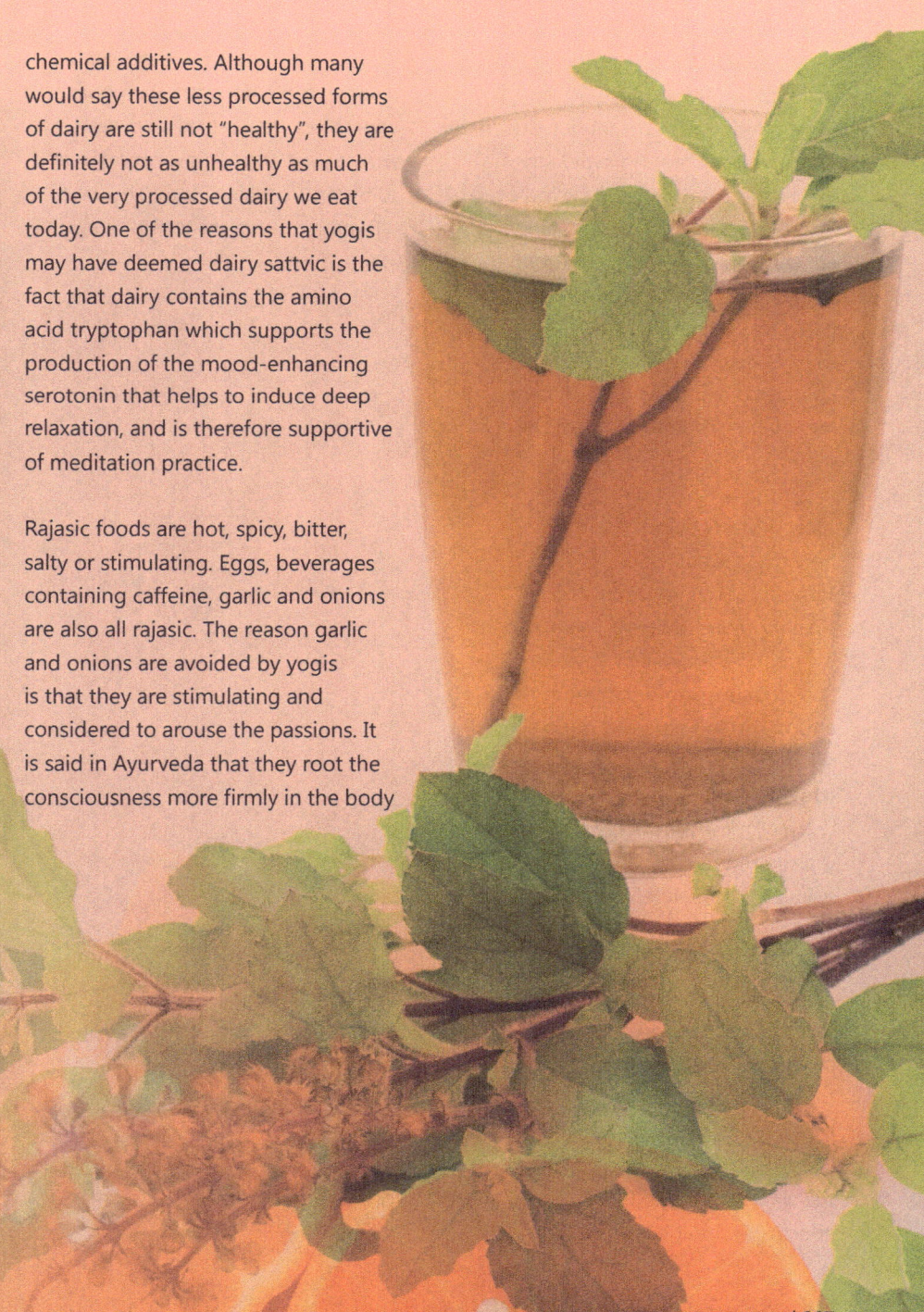

chemical additives. Although many would say these less processed forms of dairy are still not "healthy", they are definitely not as unhealthy as much of the very processed dairy we eat today. One of the reasons that yogis may have deemed dairy sattvic is the fact that dairy contains the amino acid tryptophan which supports the production of the mood-enhancing serotonin that helps to induce deep relaxation, and is therefore supportive of meditation practice.

Rajasic foods are hot, spicy, bitter, salty or stimulating. Eggs, beverages containing caffeine, garlic and onions are also all rajasic. The reason garlic and onions are avoided by yogis is that they are stimulating and considered to arouse the passions. It is said in Ayurveda that they root the consciousness more firmly in the body and are deemed to be both rajasic and tamasic. Bland foods are much more conducive to meditation, which is why yogis choose to avoid any foods that might make the mind over-active. These days garlic and onions are usually considered to be good for us, acting as natural antibiotics. Many herbs and spices have been shown to have phenomenal health benefits. So unless you are on a meditation retreat, it is recommended to eat them.

Alcohol starts out as rajasic but becomes tamasic once consumed. Tamasic food is all "dead" food such as processed food, meat, fish, mushrooms, sugar and any fermented foods. Stale, overripe or under-ripe, and/or rotten foods and the practice of over-eating are also tamasic. For yogis abiding by the yamas and niyamas meat is not only tamasic, it is also prohibited by the first yama, ahimsa or non-violence.

In keeping with this shunning of meat *The China Study*, the biggest scientific study of nutrition ever undertaken, proves beyond a shadow of a doubt that consumption of animal products, including dairy, causes heart disease and cancer. Based on this book, the film *Forks Over Knives* is very informative on the subject.

To conclude, today the best diet for a yogi is high in fresh raw organic vegetables, vegetable juices, sprouts and soaked nuts. This is considered to be the healthiest option by most alternative nutritionists these days.

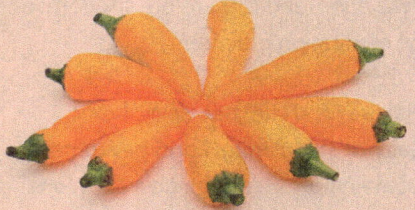

"What we eat not only affects how we look physically, but also how we feel and how clear and creative our mental energy is. Some foods support and enliven our yoga practice and life-force energy, whilst other foods inhibit and undermine them."

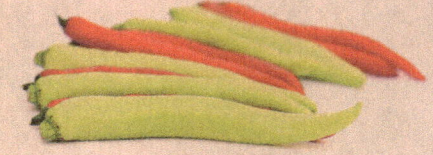

SNOWFLAKES – Water

Water descending from the Sky has a purifying effect on Earth –and yes, it can also have a devastating effect! From a cosmic perspective, rain often represents an energy flow from a higher to a lower place. This flow of water can slow down so much as to acquire a solid form, as in the case of snow, which is formed of tiny ice crystals or snowflakes. A white mantle of snow on a winter's day speaks of cleanliness and makes everything "equal in purity". But the snowflakes are in themselves totally individual. As they fall to the ground through the atmosphere's different temperatures and conditions of humidity, their shape of beautiful geometric patterns changes continuously. Not two of them are alike. Eventually, snowflakes melt down and turn back into flowing water, very much like the individual soul is reunited with its Source at the end of its journey.

December 2014

December 2014

1	2	3	4	5	6	7
8	9	10	11	12	13	14
15	16	17	18	19	20	21
22	23	24	25	26	27	28
29	30	31				

PLANNER HANDBOOK JOURNAL | 211

December 2014

1
MONDAY

2
TUESDAY

3
WEDNESDAY

Sutra III.48 *grahana svarupasmitanvayarthavattva*
samyamad indriya jayah

4
THURSDAY

5
FRIDAY

Full Moon ◯   **6**
SATURDAY

7
SUNDAY

December 2014

1	2	3	4	5	6	7	week 49
8	9	10	11	12	13	14	
15	16	17	18	19	20	21	
22	23	24	25	26	27	28	
29	30	31					

December 2014

8
MONDAY

9
TUESDAY

10
WEDNESDAY

Sutra III.49 *tato manojavitvam vikaranabhavah pradhana jayas ca*

Sutra III.50 *sattva purusanyatakhyatimatrasya sarva bhavadhisthatrtvam sarvajnatrtvam ca*

December 2014

11
THURSDAY

12
FRIDAY

13
SATURDAY

Last Quarter  ## 14
SUNDAY

December 2014

1	2	3	4	5	6	7
8	9	10	11	12	13	14
15	16	17	18	19	20	21
22	23	24	25	26	27	28
29	30	31				

week 50

December 2014

15
MONDAY

16
TUESDAY

17
WEDNESDAY

Sutra III.51 *tad vairagyad api dosa bija ksaye kaivalyam*

Sutra III.52 *sthanyupanimantrane sanga smayakaranam*
                    punar anista prasangat

18
THURSDAY

19
FRIDAY

20
SATURDAY

21
SUNDAY

December 2014

1	2	3	4	5	6	7
8	9	10	11	12	13	14
15	16	17	18	19	20	21
22	23	24	25	26	27	28
29	30	31				

week 51

December 2014

22 New Moon
MONDAY   Winter Solstice

23
TUESDAY

24
WEDNESDAY

Sutra III.53 *ksana tat kramayoh samyamad vivekajam jnanam*

Sutra III.54 *jati laksana desair anyatanavacchedat tulyayos tatah pratipattih*

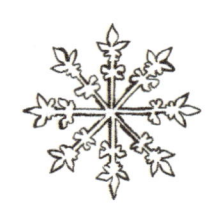

25
THURSDAY

26
FRIDAY

27
SATURDAY

First Quarter **28**
SUNDAY

December 2014

1	2	3	4	5	6	7
8	9	10	11	12	13	14
15	16	17	18	19	20	21
22	23	24	25	26	27	28
29	30	31

week 52

December 2014

29
MONDAY

30
TUESDAY

31
WEDNESDAY

Sutra III.55 *tarakam sarva visayam sarvatha visayam akraman ceti vivekajam jnanam*

Sutra III.56 *sattva pursayoh suddhi samye kaivalyam*

1
THURSDAY

2
FRIDAY

3
SATURDAY

4
SUNDAY

December 2014

1	2	3	4	5	6	7
8	9	10	11	12	13	14
15	16	17	18	19	20	21
22	23	24	25	26	27	28
29	30	31				

week 1

SQUAT
Kidney Meridian

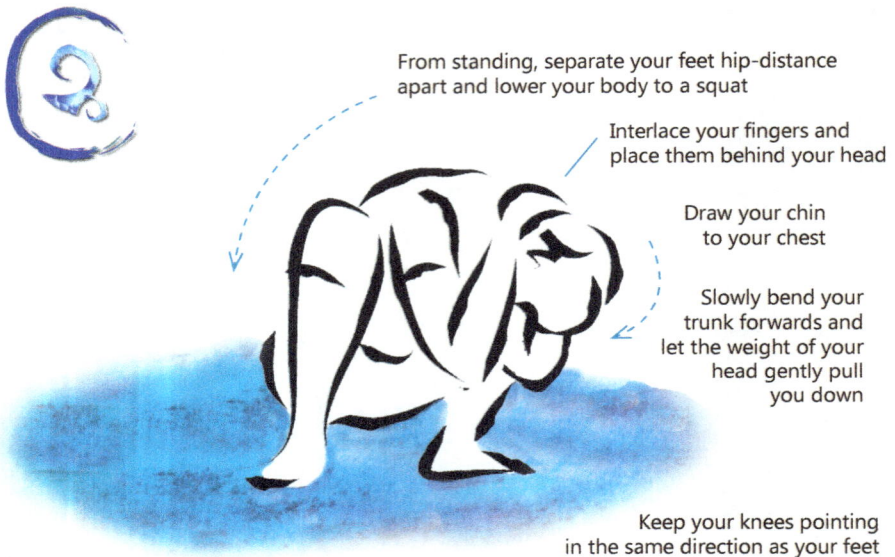

From standing, separate your feet hip-distance apart and lower your body to a squat

Interlace your fingers and place them behind your head

Draw your chin to your chest

Slowly bend your trunk forwards and let the weight of your head gently pull you down

Keep your knees pointing in the same direction as your feet

While in the Pose
- Holding time: 2 to 3 minutes.
- Breathe deeply and mindfully.

Coming out of the Pose
- Leave the pose slowly and mindfully.
- Place your hands flat on the ground in front of you. Inhale and raise your hips. Exhale and fall forwards into Uttanasana (Standing Forward Bend) with your knees slightly bent.
- Observe the effects of the pose.

Modifications and Variations
- If your heels are not touching the ground, place a rolled-up blanket or block under them.
- Feel free to change the position of your feet to avoid painful compression in your groins.

Taking it Further
- Bring your feet closer together to further stimulate the ankles.

Meridians and Organs Affected

The Liver and Kidney meridians (groins and inner legs).
The Urinary Bladder meridian (dorsal and lumbar spine).
The Stomach meridian (ankles).
It applies healthy stress to the ovaries.

Anatomical Benefits

It opens up the hips.
It releases the dorsal and lumbar areas.
It strengthens the ankles.

Contraindications

Knee issues.

Yang Sibling

Malasana (Garland Pose). In the Yang yoga version of this pose, we keep the back straight and reaching upwards. The hands are together in Anjali Mudra (Prayer Position) and the elbows push against the inner knees to further open up the hips.

If you feel any painful sensation in your groins, use a variation of the pose!

MY NOTES

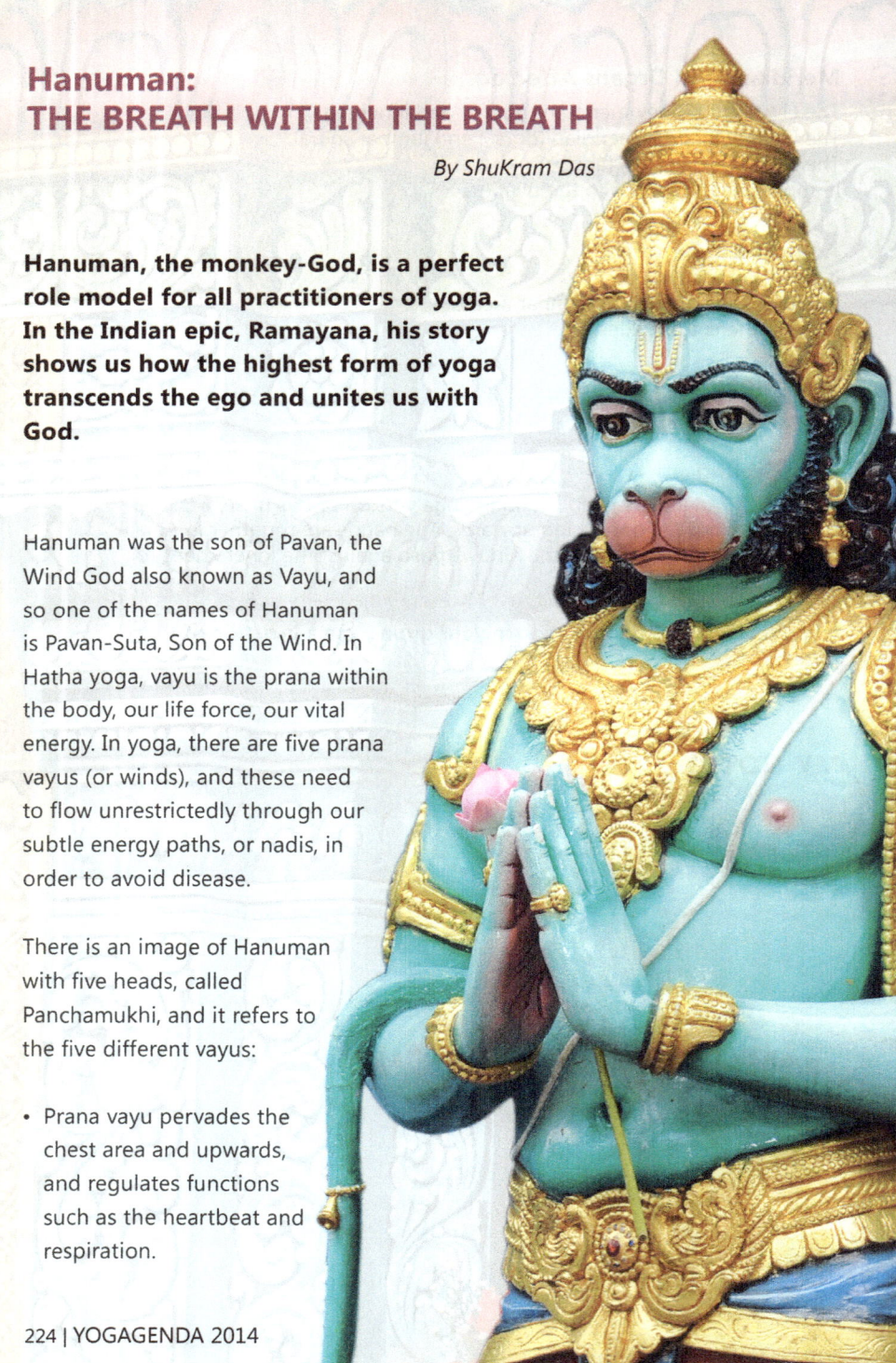

Hanuman:
THE BREATH WITHIN THE BREATH

By ShuKram Das

Hanuman, the monkey-God, is a perfect role model for all practitioners of yoga. In the Indian epic, Ramayana, his story shows us how the highest form of yoga transcends the ego and unites us with God.

Hanuman was the son of Pavan, the Wind God also known as Vayu, and so one of the names of Hanuman is Pavan-Suta, Son of the Wind. In Hatha yoga, vayu is the prana within the body, our life force, our vital energy. In yoga, there are five prana vayus (or winds), and these need to flow unrestrictedly through our subtle energy paths, or nadis, in order to avoid disease.

There is an image of Hanuman with five heads, called Panchamukhi, and it refers to the five different vayus:

• Prana vayu pervades the chest area and upwards, and regulates functions such as the heartbeat and respiration.

- Apana vayu pervades the area from the navel and downwards and regulates urination, menstrual cycle and giving birth, among other functions of elimination.
- Samana vayu pervades the area between the navel and heart where yoga is the union of prana and apana, and it regulates digestion, assimilation of food, etc.
- Udana vayu pervades the head area and regulates functions such as the blinking of the eyes, coughing, hiccups, and sneezing.
- Vyana vayu circulates throughout the body in all directions.

Prana is different from breath. Breath is the tool to work with prana, to control and direct it through breathing techniques or pranayamas that help discipline the mind. Breath and mind are very much interlinked. When the mind is upset, angry, lustful, etc. the breath will be fast; when the mind is calm, the breath will be calm also. As the mind influences the breath, you can also influence the mind with the breath.

In the Ramayana, the world's oldest poem written by Valmiki, Hanuman acts as the mediator between Rama (God) and his wife Sita (the individual soul). Sita is kidnapped by Ravana (the ego) and separated from Rama. Captured in the world of temptation, she experiences fear and anxiety and almost loses the will to live. At the moment when she is in her darkest hour, Hanuman manifests himself and gives her a token of hope and a message that there is an eternal chord of love between God and the individual soul. All Sita needs to do is keep her faith and concentrate her mind on God.

By remembering Rama (God), Hanuman revived his own hidden strength and was able to do the impossible: jump over the ocean to Lanka, find Sita and help kill all the demons. Despite Hanuman's strength and power, he is a perfectly humble servant, remembering always that he is not primarily the doer of action. He didn't perform any action for fame or gain. When you practise yoga just for self-interest, you're only boosting your ego (ravana), leading to destruction. Hanuman shows us that the highest yoga is to always remember Rama (God). In this way he is the perfect example of a karma yogi.

In yoga it is the breath and devotion that reunites us back with God as well.

Hanuman is the breath within the breath.

He is aware of his breath all the time. We inhale and exhale mostly without much awareness, but for Hanuman every inhalation is about receiving grace and every exhalation about surrender and giving devotion. We should appreciate the value of each breath. We only know the worth of the breath when we are on our last breath!

Hanuman is especially worshipped on Tuesdays and Saturdays, days that are associated with Mars and Saturn. To invoke the powers of Hanuman, devotees sing the Hanuman Chalisa, a hymn of 40 verses written by the poet Tulsidas in the 16th century. There is also reference in the work to Hanuman being

the bestower of the eight siddhis or powers that are described in the third chapter of Patanjali's Yoga Sutras*, as well as the nine ways of devotion. The Hanuman Chalisa is said to bring peace into the devotee's life along with wealth, strength, fearlessness, ecstasy and ultimately offer liberation from worldly things.

*Mangala Murati Maruta Nandana,
Sakala Amangala Mula Nikandana
Son of the Wind, embodiment of all
blessings, you destroy the root of all
that is harmful and inauspicious.*

* Featured weekly in this edition of
Yogagenda and translated into English
on our website.

"When you practise yoga just for self-interest, you're only boosting your ego (ravana), leading to destruction. Hanuman shows us that the highest yoga is to always remember Rama (God). In this way he is the perfect example of a karma yogi."

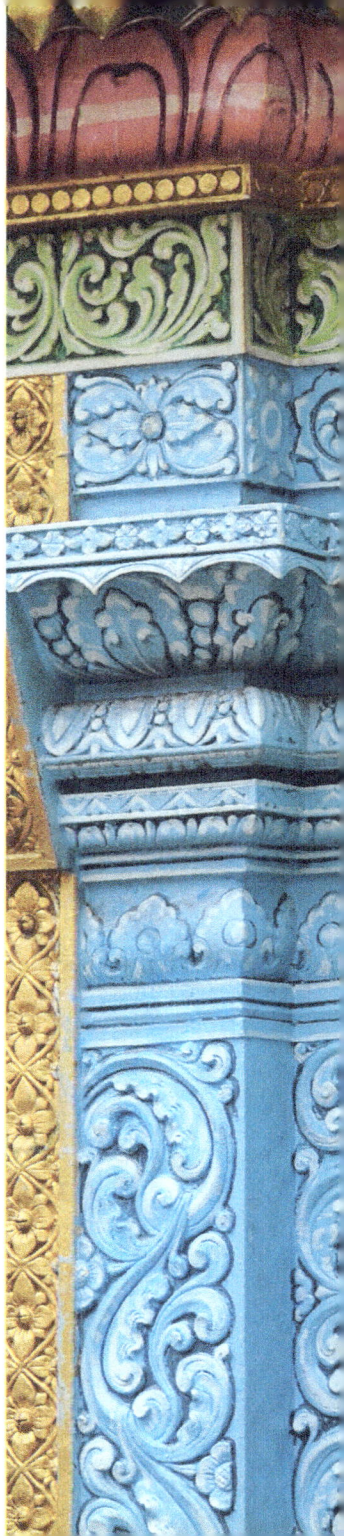

The Sequence:
YIN FOR THE SPINE

By Mariah Mansvelt Beck

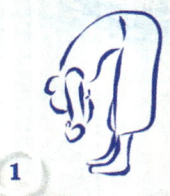

1

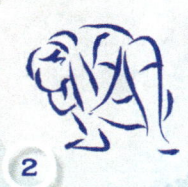

2

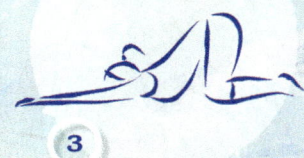

3

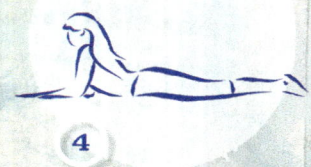

4

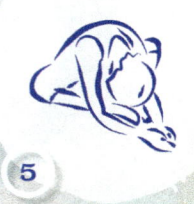

5

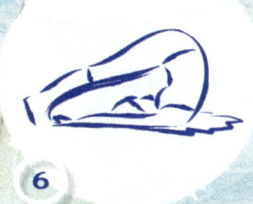

6

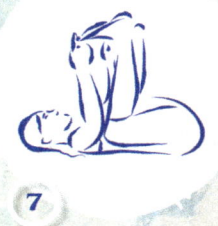

7

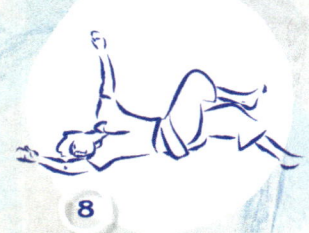

8

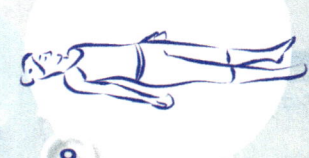

9

This sequence focuses on stretching and stimulating the entire spine in a slow and mindful manner. Lose your ambition and just allow your body to take its time to slowly unwind in each pose. Be mindful of how your pose evolves. If you lose the sensation, see if you can deepen your pose. If the pose becomes a struggle (in your mind and/or your body!) see if you can soften your breath, which may in turn help to soften your body as well as your mind. If need be, back off.

1 DANGLING

Stand with both feet hip-distance apart. Slowly roll down vertebrae by vertebrae. Hold your opposite elbow with your hand if you want. To focus more on releasing your lower back, bend your knees; to focus more on the hamstrings, keep the legs straight.

Holding time: 3 minutes.

> **Counterpose**: Slowly bend your knees and come directly into a squat.

2 SQUAT

Take your feet wide apart (place a roll under your heels if they don't make it to the ground). Interlace your fingers and place them behind your head drawing your chin to your chest. Slowly bend your trunk forwards and let the weight of your head gently pull you down.

Holding time: 2 minutes.

> **Counterpose**: Stretch out your legs for a minute, then come back through squat to Balasana (Child's Pose).

3 ANAHATASANA

From Balasana bring your buttocks approximately over your knees, while walking your hands forwards. Allow your forehead to rest on the ground and focus on the stretch in your upper and middle back as well as your shoulders. If you want to go deeper, try resting your chin on the ground. If you are struggling, rest your forehead on a block or bend your arms instead of keeping them straight.

Holding time: 3 minutes.

> **Counterpose**: Rest in Balasana for a minute.

4 SPHINX AND SEAL

Come to lie on your stomach and bring your elbows approximately under your shoulders. Allow your trunk to sink between your shoulders and feel free to allow your neck to hang or to keep it at neutral. If you want to deepen the pose, take your hands a little out to the sides and straighten your arms for Seal. If your lower back is sensitive, you can always bring your elbows further forwards or even rest your head on your hands or a folded blanket.

Holding time: 4 minutes.

> **Counterpose**: First rest your forehead on your hands lying down. When you're ready push yourself back and rest in a wide-legged Balasana, so that your spine can rest in between your legs.

5 BUTTERFLY

Bring your feet together a bit further apart than you would normally do in an active yoga practice, and make a diamond shape with your legs. Slowly allow yourself to roll down. You can always place props under your thighs if the stretch becomes too much. If you start to build up too much tension in your head or neck, try lifting your head a little until you can relax it down again.

Holding time: 5 minutes.

> **Counterpose**: Slowly come out of the pose and use your arms to bring your knees back up. Rest back on your elbows and allow your knees to fall from one side to the other for around a minute to neutralise the spine.

6 SNAIL

Lying down on the ground, slowly bring your legs overhead, and aim to bring your feet to the ground behind you. If your feet don't touch the ground, use your arms on your lower back to support yourself and feel free to rest your knees on your forehead. If your feet touch the ground you can take your outstretched arms towards your feet. If you want to deepen the posture, you can bend your knees until they close off your ears.

While in this pose it is important not to move your neck from side to side. You should also not experience pressure on your cervical (neck) vertebrae. If you do, see if you can come more onto your shoulder blades by moving

these further under yourself, or by using a folded blanket and placing it so it is in line with your shoulders allowing more space for your neck.
Holding time: 3 minutes.

> **Counterpose:** Slowly roll out of the posture and come to lie on the ground, feeling the effects of this extreme forward bend. After about a minute, bring your knees into your chest and make small circles with your knees. If you need to release tension in your upper or middle back, bring your neck up to your knees for a little while.

7   STIRRUP

Part your knees and take hold of your toes, feet, ankles or the back of your feet/thighs with your hands. By allowing your tailbone to lift off the ground there is the opportunity to release the sacroiliac joints. Pulling further with your hands will move your knees closer to the ground, helping to open up your hips. If your hamstrings are under too much pressure, feel free to bring your feet towards your buttocks.
Holding time: 2 minutes.

> **Counterpose:** Slowly release your feet, bring your knees together, take hold of your knees with your hands and make small circles to massage your lower back into the ground.

8   RECLINING TWIST

Finish your practice with a twist. Bring your legs further up towards your chest if you want to target your lower spine, or bring your legs in line with or lower than your hips if you want to target your sacrum region and hips.
Holding time: 2 minutes on each side.

> **Counterpose:** Slowly make your way into the final relaxation pose. If your lower spine feels sensitive, you can always hold your knees to your chest for a minute or keep your knees bent (with a bolster under your knees) during the final relaxation.

9   SAVASANA

Relax and integrate your practice. Take the time for your body to neutralise and be mindful of the flow of energy throughout it. Stay for at least 2 minutes, but feel free to extend.

Yoga Festivals & Celebrations Around The Globe

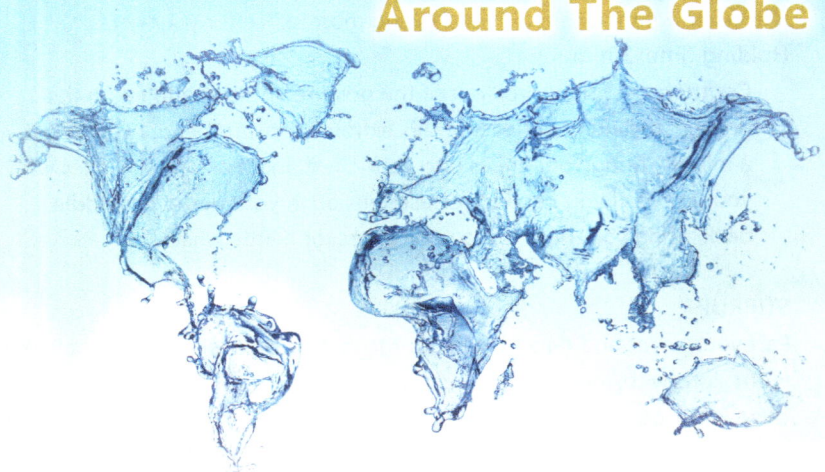

Compiled by Michelle Taffe from <u>theglobalyogi.com</u>. For up-to-date information on all of these events, please check <u>http://calendar.theglobalyogi.com/events/category/festivals/</u>

JANUARY

**Yoga Journal Conference:
San Francisco (California, USA)**
Four days of yoga with classes in all styles for all levels.
<u>www.yjevents.com/sf14</u>

**Kundalini Yoga Festival
(San Esteban, Chile)**
Six days of Kundalini yoga practice, expanding on the teachings of Yogi Bhajan in the mighty Chilean Andes.
<u>www.kundaliniyogafestival.cl</u>

**Texas Yoga Conference
(Houston, USA)**
Three days to learn and practise yoga with prominent Texan and national teachers. "Om in the heart of Texas."
<u>www.texasyogaconference.com</u>

FEBRUARY

**Austria Yoga Conference
(Wels, Austria)**
Three days celebrating yoga in Wels, a pretty town on the Traun river in northern Austria.
<u>www.yoga-conference.at</u>

**Caribbean Yoga Conference
(Montego Bay, Jamaica)**
Four days celebrating sadhana, sand, seva and sangha under the sun in the Caribbean.
<u>www.caribbeanyogaconference.com</u>

**Olis Festival
(Milan, Italy)**
Two days dedicated to the innate wellness of the body, mind and spirit in Milan.
<u>www.olisfestival.it</u>

Wanderlust Festival
(Chile)
Three days to share yoga in a spa hotel in Chile together with great yoga teachers, musicians, artists and performers.
chile.wanderlustfestival.com

Chant Fest
(Denver, USA)
Three days of chanting in Denver, Colorado with the world's best conscious music and yoga instructors.
denverchantfest.com

Wanderlust Festival
(Oahu, USA)
Four days to share yoga by the surf in Hawaii –"Your yoga mat just grew a fin!"– together with great yoga teachers, musicians, artists and performers.
oahu.wanderlustfestival.com

MARCH

Byron Spirit Festival
(Byron Bay, Australia)
Three days of yoga, music, tantra and dance in beautiful Mullumbimby in Byron Shire, Australia.
www.spiritfestival.com.au

Canon Beach Yoga Festival
(Oregon, USA)
Three days of yoga, art, health, wellness treatments, spa and fun on the Pacific Northwest coast.
www.cannonbeachyogafestival.com

International Yoga Festival
(Rishikesh, India)
Seven days on the banks of the sacred river Ganga; a week-long celebration of yoga and one of the world's largest yoga events. Learn from the best of India's spiritual leaders.
www.internationalyogafestival.com

BaliSpirit Festival
(Bali, Indonesia)
Five days of yoga workshops, concerts, healing and community magnified by the magical spirit of Bali.
www.balispiritfestival.com

SpiritFest
(Cape Town, South Africa)
Three days of yoga, dance and music in the grounds of a beautiful winery estate not far from Cape Town. Get ready to have your heart opened wide!
www.spiritfest.co.za

Yoga Festival
(Catania, Italy)
Three days over a weekend completely dedicated to finding harmony through yoga practice in Sicily.
www.yogafestival.it

Yoga Art Festival Mexico
(Amecameca, Mexico)
Eight days of awakening, exploring the potential of human creativity and yoga in the foothills of a sacred volcano.
www.yogaartfestival.com

Bodhi Festival
(Newcastle, Australia)
Three days of yoga, healing and music in this coastal Australian city.
www.bodhifestival.com.au

APRIL

Yoga Journal Conference: New York (New York, USA)
Five days of yoga with classes in all styles and for all levels.
www.yjevents.com/ny14

Evolve Yoga and Wellness Festival (Melbourne, Australia)
A one-day coming together of the southern hemisphere yoga and wellness community.
www.evolveyogafestival.com.au

MAY

Yoga and Holistic Europe (Merano, Italy)
Two days over a weekend completely dedicated to finding harmony through yoga practice in the South Tyrol.
http://www.yogameeting.org/

British Kundalini Yoga Festival (Reading, England)
Six days of yoga in a friendly, nurturing environment of joy, devotion and service to all beings, rooted in the Kundalini yoga teachings of Yogi Bhajan.
www.kundaliniyogafestival.org.uk

Midsummer Festival of Yoga (Dorset, England)
Four days of "celebrating diversity in yoga" with workshops, discussions, music, dance and more in the English countryside.
www.yogafestival.org.uk

German Yoga Conference (Cologne, Germany)
Four days to "find freedom" in Cologne, at one of the most established yoga gatherings in Europe.
www.yogaconference.de

JUNE

Bhakti Yoga Summer (Bad Staffelstein, Germany)
Three days of love, yoga and music in the Bavarian countryside. Join in celebrating the "flowering of the heart".
bhaktiyogasummer.com

Evolution Asia Yoga Conference (Hong Kong, China)
Four days of yoga in Hong Kong at Asia's largest annual yoga and wellness conference serving the growing interest in yoga in the region.
www.asiayogaconference.com

Berlin Yoga Festival (Berlin, Germany)
Three days to cherish "every breath you take" of yoga outdoors – at the Kladow Cultural Park.
www.yogafestival.de

Hanuman Festival (Colorado, USA)
Four days to honour the beauty of yoga and music in this community-oriented festival at the foot of Colorado's Rocky Mountains.
www.hanumanfestival.com

**Wanderlust Festival
(Vermont, USA)**
Four days to share yoga with the world's leading yoga teachers, musicians and DJs, speakers, chefs and winemakers!
stratton.wanderlustfestival.com

**Dutch Yoga Festival
(Terschelling, The Netherlands)**
Three days immersed in yoga on a Dutch island; enjoying beaches, camping, lake swimming, cycling and more.
www.yogafestival.info

**Brisbane Yoga Fest
(Brisbane, Australia)**
Two days to connect, discover and celebrate at Australia's largest and longest-running celebration of yoga.
www.yogafest.com.au

JULY

**Wanderlust Festival
(Colorado, USA)**
Four days to share yoga in rural Colorado together with great yoga teachers, musicians, artists and performers.
colorado.wanderlustfestival.com

**Barcelona Yoga Conference
(Barcelona, Spain)**
Five days of inspiration in Barcelona with a team of renowned and dedicated teachers offering their personal vision of ancient yogic wisdom.
www.barcelonayogaconference.cat

**Colourfest
(Dorset, England)**
Three days to glam it up in elegant tents while celebrating life through yoga, music and dance in Dorset.
colourfest.co.uk

**Bliss Beat Festival
(Sezzadio, Italy)**
Four days in the Italian countryside sharing the magic of yoga and devotional kirtan.
www.blissbeatfestival.com

**Telluride Festival
(Colorado, USA)**
Four days in the small Colorado mountain town of Telluride to share the teachings of yoga. This is a zero waste festival.
tellurideyogafestival.com

**Nantucket Yoga Festival
(Massachusetts, USA)**
Three days to celebrate yoga, health and wellness on the island of Nantucket off the east coast of North America.
nantucketyogafestival.com

**Ängsbacka Yoga Festival
(Molkom, Sweden)**
Seven days in the Nordic countryside focusing on ahimsa – bringing peace and freedom to yourself and the world – with yoga enthusiasts of all levels and traditions.
uk.angsbacka.se

**Wanderlust Festival
(California, USA)**
Four days of fantastic yoga, healing, music, hiking and more near the serene Lake Tahoe in California.
squaw.wanderlustfestival.com

**European Yoga Festival
(Fondjouan, France)**
Nine days of Kundalini yoga following the teachings of Yogi Bhajan – in a fairytale-like French chateau in a forest! Swim in one of two lakes on the property in between yoga sessions!
www.3ho-kundalini-yoga.eu

AUGUST

**Wanderlust Festival
(Whistler, Canada)**
Four days of fantastic yoga, healing, music, hiking and more in the mountains of Whistler in Canada.
whistler.wanderlustfestival.com

**International Yoga and Ayurveda Conference
(Sao Paulo, Brazil)**
Five days of yoga, Ayurveda and music at Sao Paulo's Parque do Ibirapuera.
www.yogapelapaz.com.br

**Wakeup Festival
(Colorado, USA)**
Five days to gather together and wake up with yogis, musicians, healers in Estes Park, Colorado.
www.wakeupfestival.com

**Finger Lakes Yoga Festival
(Ithaca, USA)**
Four days to celebrate yoga, music and art in stunning countryside of Ithaca, in New York State.
www.fingerlakesyogafestival.org

**NavaNadi Yoga Festival
(Belgium)**
Three-day festival of yoga, music and meditation in the Belgian countryside.
navanadifestival.com

SEPTEMBER

**Geneva Yoga Music Festival
(Geneva, Switzerland)**
Five glorious days in the heart of the city, near the lake and parks. A cool and peaceful celebration of music, yoga, massage and other surprises.
www.genevayogamusicfestival.ch

**Evolve Yoga and Wellness Festival
(Sydney, Australia)**
Two days for the coming together of the southern hemisphere yoga and wellness community on Sydney Harbour.
www.evolveyogafestival.com.au/

**Bhakti Fest West
(Joshua Tree, USA)**
Four days celebrating devotion through music, chanting, yoga, meditation and community in California desert.
www.bhaktifest.com

**Kindred Spirit Festival
(Melbourne, Australia)**
Two days celebrating music, movement and meditation with a global view for peace and prosperity.
www.kindredspiritfest.com

**Ibiza Yoga Festival
(Spain)**
Three days of sun, sea and yoga in the Spanish Mediterranean on the island of Ibiza, when the late summer sun is still warm.
www.yogafestival.info/ibiza

Annual Yoga Journal Conference: Colorado (USA)
Seven days of yoga with classes in all styles and for all levels.
www.yjevents.com/ep

OCTOBER

**Freiburg Yoga and Music Festival
(Germany)**
Three days to come together to share
yoga and music in Germany. Inspired
by the community spirit of Auroville.
www.freiburgyogamusikfestival.de

**Kundalini Yoga Asia Festival
(Thailand)**
13 days dedicated to serve, inspire
and empower humanity to be healthy,
happy and whole through the
teachings of Kundalini yoga in Thailand.
www.kundaliniyogaasia.org

**Divine Play AcroYoga Festival
(Portland, USA)**
Four days of divine play with
Acroyoga and many other special
events in Oregon.
www.acroyoga.org/acroyogafestival

**Iowa City Yoga Festival
(Iowa, USA)**
Three days of yoga, music and fun
held in this Midwest location.
www.iowacityyogafestival.com

**Austin Yoga Festival
(Texas, USA)**
Two days to come celebrate the traditions of yoga with Austin's finest yoga
teachers, presenters and musicians.
www.austinyogafestival.com

**Yoga Festival
(Milan, Italy)**
Three days over a weekend
completely dedicated to finding
harmony through yoga practice in
Milan.
www.yogafestival.it

**Ojai Yoga Crib
(California, USA)**
Four days of yoga in the Ojai Valley
in California - a magical spot long
regarded as a place for spiritual
pilgrimage.
www.lulubandhas.com/yoga/crib

**Yoga Journal Conference:
Florida (USA)**
Four days of yoga with classes in all
styles and for all levels.
www.yjevents.com/florida

NOVEMBER

**Dubai Yoga and Music Festival
(Dubai, UAE)**
Three days of yoga, music and
meditation in the Middle East: Shakti
in the dunes – fruits of the desert!
www.dubaiyogafest.com

**Namaste Festival
(Jakarta, Indonesia)**
Three days of yoga in Jakarta.
Discover your potential, explore
different yoga styles and connect with
local and international yogis.
www.namastefestival.com

Who Contributed To Yogagenda 2014

A hearth-felt thank you to all the great people who have contributed in different ways to the making of this Yogagenda, whether it's been with inspiring editorial contributions or great artwork, with helpful marketing advice, with creative graphic/web design or with careful copy editing and proofreading, and in many other ways. While putting together this issue, I've realised we all have something very important in common: passion for what we do. I hope it is contagious and that you, reader, enjoy using your copy as much as I did putting it together. Thanks for walking this path with us!

Elena

Elena Sepúlveda

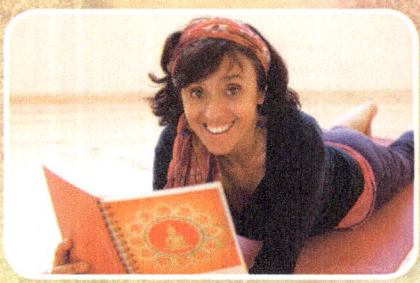

As founder, publisher and editor of *Yogagenda*, Elena is the beating heart of this project that brings together her love for yoga and her passion for publishing. She is a qualified yoga teacher (Vinyasa and Yin) and body worker (Chavutti Thirumal and Thai massage), but also a published writer and translator. Her aim is to creatively blend both facets, finding enjoyable and beneficial ways to share the results.

Seed-Joy.com

Martin Aylward (The Body of Life). Martin has been immersed in meditation practice since 1989, spending five years in Asian monasteries and with Himalayan hermits before founding his own centre, Moulin de Chaves, in South West France. He teaches meditation and leads retreats worldwide, emphasising a creative approach to awakening in all aspecats of life.
MoulindeChaves.org
MartinAylward.com

Wenche Beard (Yoga in the First Person).
Born in Norway and trained with the British Wheel of Yoga, Wenche is the founder and director of the Yoga-Life Studio in Eastbourne, England. Through her yoga teachings she helps others to live bravely, joyfully and passionately, to free themselves from barriers and restrictions, so they can be true to who they really are. She runs retreats and offers a unique and fun-filled Yoga Teacher Training program.
Yoga-Life.co.uk
YogaLifeRetreats.co.uk

Sarah Dawson (The Koshas).
Journalist & author, Sarah, trained as a Sivananda yoga teacher in 2007 and began teaching in 2008. Following her intuition she undertook a further 200-hour training in Dru Yoga and now teaches a flowing synthesis of both styles, with emphasis on "internalising" the benefits of yoga. She is author of Everyday Yoga: The Essential Guide and continues to write regularly for travel/well-being publications.
KarmiYoga.com

Gabrielle Green (Copy Editing).
Yoga has been an on-again, off-again feature in Gabrielle's life since 1990. Although she's been more "yogi–no" than "yogi–ni" recently, she plans to populate Yogagenda 2014 with more time for yoga and self. Barcelona-based and Australian-born, she takes on publishing projects, teaches English and continues to explore her new city when not chasing after toddler Xavi.
gabrielle@yogagendas.com

José de Groot (Yin & Yan Yoga).
José has been teaching mainly Yin but also Hatha, Vinyasa and Vini yoga since 2006, after having completed a 200-hour Yoga Teacher Training in Barcelona. Since then she continues her yoga studies with teachers all over the world, such as Paul Grilley, Sarah Powers and T.K.V. Desikachar. She currently offers weekly classes, workshops, Yin Yoga & Anatomy Teacher Trainings and retreats in The Netherlands, Spain, Finland and France.
YogaTreat.eu

Vidya Heisel (To Eat or Not to Eat).
Vidya is a Yoga Teacher Trainer, who has been studying and practising yoga for 37 years. She is the Director of Frog Lotus Yoga International and runs Yoga Teacher Training programs around the world in exctic locations, as well as at her beloved home retreat centre, Suryalila Retreat Centre in Andalusia, Spain. Vidya is also the creator of Envision Yoga.
FrogLotusYogaInternational.com

David Lurey (Mantra and Vibration).
David is a passionate musician and yogi who shares these important facets of personal deve opment through trainings, workshops and musical offerings around the world.

His chanting and music lifts the spirits of all who share the space with him and he has self-produced two mantra CDs to balance the dedicated and disciplined asana practice that he also loves to share.
FindBalance.net
davidlurey.bandcamp.com/album/global-bhakti-project

Mariah Mansvelt Beck (Yin Sequence for the Spine).
Mariah is a yoga teacher in the Amsterdam area. In perhaps a familiar search for happiness, stress relief and balance she has, time and time again, returned to her yoga practice and is grateful for the opportunity to share this with others. She teaches both active Vinyasa as well as quiet Yin yoga. For an overview of her classes, check
delightyoga.nl
yogamoves.nl
sukhayoga.nl

Marta Moia (Monthly Symbols illustrations).
Marta trained as a painter at art school in her native Buenos Aires. Later she studied Textile Design at Chelsea School of Art in London, where she spent many years working in the arts and publishing before moving to southern Spain. She continues painting and taking inspiration from her surroundings in the mountains of Las Alpujarras, Granada.

Irantzu Piquero (The Goddess of a Thousand Faces).
Irantzu is a yoga teacher and also holds a Literature Degree. Always fascinated with the connection between image and word, she shares the potential of storytelling as a transformational vehicle, decoding

Indian teachings through their most popular and graphic aspects: mythology and art. Her classes and workshops are inspired by the Rajanaka Tantra teachings, within the Sri Vidya tradition.
YogayMitologia.com

Swami Saradananda (Meditation).
An internationally-renowned yoga–meditation teacher, she is the author of many books including *Chakra Meditation*, *Power of Breath*, *Yoga Mind and Body*, *Relax and Unwind with Yoga*, and *Essential Guide to Chakras*. After working with Sivananda Yoga Centres for many years, she did intensive personal practice in the Himalayas. Now based in London, she teaches worldwide, including the popular 3-month programme for yoga teachers: "Teach Meditation".
FlyingMountainYoga.org

Michelle Taffe (Yoga Festivals & Celebrations).
Michelle is the founder of the digital yoga hub The Global Yogi – comprising a Yogazine, a monthly News Digest and an Event Calendar – which connects yogis with teachers, studios, retreat centres and yoga events worldwide. A yogi and a writer with a background in web design, Michelle is now based in Australia, but has lived most of the last 10 years in Spain.
TheGlobalYogi.com

Denise Ullmann (*Yogagenda*'s logo; Illustrations for Asanas and The Sequence).
Born in Buenos Aires, she practises yoga, acroyoga, dancing, and most of all she has painted for as long as she can remember. After studying arts, Denise has worked in a variety

of projects such as illustrating logos for festivals, postcards, CD covers and stories. She has also edited her first own illustrated book, Asai Va.
AbriendoUnMundo.blogspot.com

ShukRam Das (Hanuman).
ShukRam Das (Patrick Vermeulen) is co-founder of SvahaYoga in Amsterdam. He teaches asana, pranayama, yoga-philosophy, meditation and chanting. He learned the Hanuman Chalisa when first travelling to India in 1999. Currently a life-size Hanuman murti has arrived from India bringing life to the new SvahaYoga Shala in Surinam.
svahayoga.com
cdbaby.com/cd/shukramdas

Mirjam Wagner (Fascia).
As an osteopath and yoga teacher, Mirjam focuses on transmitting the knowledge of human anatomy in a simple, transparent and very efficient way. She brings new understanding of body, mind and soul to yoga practice and to daily life habits to support the inherent healing process. Mirjam offers courses all over Europe and runs teacher trainings and immersions together with her husband David Lurey.
YogaTherapyMallorca.com

Sue Woodd and Julie Hanson
(Seasonal Energy).
Sue and Julie have been working in the field of seasonal living and yoga for over 15 years. A book, 5 seasonal DVD's, and an online seasonal training course (as a bolt-on for qualified teachers), plus a full year 200-hour YA teacher training are some of the products available from them at
SeasonalYoga.co.uk
EnergyYogaSchool.com

Artist as stated below/Shutterstock.com
Front cover image: Andrea Haase
Inside pages: katatonia82 (pp.2-3), Andrea Haase (pp.4-7), Iwona Grodzka (pp.8-9), Jakez (pp.10-11), Elena Ray (p.12; p.27; p.58; pp.72-75; pp.228-231; pp. 248-249; pp.253-254; pp. 257-258; pp.261-262), Adam Rauso (p.13; p.45), Madlen (p.14; p.61), sevenke (p.15; p.77), szefei (p.16; p.95), Floydine (p.17; p.111), Agnieszka Barbara (p.18; p.127), Andrea Haase (p.19; p.145), Jiří Hodecek (p.20; p.161), Franziska Lang (p.21; p.177), Stephen VanHorn (p.22; p.195), elwynn (p.23; p.211), Larissa Kulik (pp.24-25), Photosani (p.24), naqib (pp. 39, 55, 71, 89, 105, 121, 139, 155, 171, 189, 205, 233), stock09 (pp.40-43), argus (pp.106-108), mario babu (p.109), Pikoso.kz (pp.122-124), shooarts (p.125), Sebastian Kaulitzki (p.174), Kjpargeter (p.175), Arman Zender (p.226), Vibrant Image Studio (pp.232-237), J.D.S. (pp.232-237), Ngo Thye Aun (pp.238-241), Ieoks (pp.242-245), kentoh (pp.242-244), uspenskava (pp.246-247), sabri deniz kizil (pp. 261-262).

Artist as stated below/Dreamstime.com
Byheaven87 (pp.56-57, 59), Ajijchan (pp.156-159), Lucelucelu... (p.207), Mjutabor (p.209), Sunsetman (pp.224-227).

Artist as stated below/Fotolia.com
Alx (p.156), adimas (pp.172-173), Irochka (p.232).

Other artists
Lucie François (pp.90-93), Roland Wimbush (p.93), Renan Kinza Mercato (pp.140-143), Sarah Sutton (pp.190-193), Nicky Thomas LRPS/nxphoto.co.uk (p.191), Min Thu/hongkiat.com (pp.206-208), ArsGrafik (pp.249, 253, 257-258).

Sanskrit Glossary

Agni: fire.

Ahimsa: non-violence; one of the five yamas within Patanjali's eight-limbed path of yoga.

Ajna: sixth chakra, or "third eye" chakra, located between the eyebrows.

Amrita: lit. "immortality"; often referred to in sacred texts as the elixir or nectar of the deities.

Anandamaya kosha: lit. "sheath made of bliss"; it corresponds to the more subtle or spiritual body.

Annamaya kosha: lit. "food sheath"; it corresponds to the coarse or physical body.

Apana: descending manifestation of prana, waste.

Apana vayu: air or wind pervading the area from the navel and downwards, and regulating urination, menstrual cycle and giving birth, among other functions of elimination.

Apas: water.

Asana: pose or posture; third stage in Patanjali's eight-limbed path of yoga.

Ashram: traditionally, a spiritual hermitage or place of retreat.

Asura: in Hinduism, a group of power-seeking deities associated with the forces of chaos and in constant battle with the devas.

Ayurveda: "the knowledge of life", a traditional Indian medicine system that uses the principles of nature to maintain health and balance.

Bhagavad Gita: a sacred text, part of the Indian epic Mahabharata, where the god Krishna teaches yoga to his devotee Arjuna.

Bhakti yoga: the path of devotion; one of the four main margas or yoga paths mentioned in the Bhagavad Gita as ways to reach liberation.

Chakras: subtle energy centres at the hub of a person's being.

Daivam: it roughly translates as enrichment, opportunity and good fortune.

Deva: in Hinduism, the benevolent gods associated with a harmonious natural order and in constant battle with the asuras.

Devi: in Hinduism, the female aspect of the divine representing consciousness and bliss.

Guna: essential quality or attribute of nature. There are three gunas: sattva, rajas and tamas.

Hatha: union of the opposites, determined effort.

Karma yoga: the path of selfless service; one of the four main margas or yoga paths mentioned in the Bhagavad Gita as ways to reach liberation.

Kirtan: group chanting, usually as a call-and-response.

Koshas: the five different layers of existence in life, our "subtle" nature.

Manomaya kosha: lit. "mind stuff sheath"; it corresponds to the mind and the five sensory organs.

Mantra: sacred sound.

Nadis: subtle energy paths or channels.

Namaste: a spoken greeting or salutation commonly used in India and among yogis everywhere.

Niyama: five self-observances when relating to the inner world; second stage in Patanjali's eight-limbed path of yoga.

Patanjali: the compiler of the Yoga Sutras.

Prakriti: the manifest world, made up of three types of energies or gunas, and described in the Bhagavad Gita as "the primal force".

Prana: subtle or vital energy.

Prana vayu: air or wind pervading the chest area and upwards, and regulating functions such as the heartbeat and respiration.

Pranayama: breathing technique; fourth stage in Patanjali's eight-limbed path of yoga.

Pranamaya kosha: lit. "energy sheath"; it is the first layer of the subtle body.

Rajas: one of the three gunas or essential qualities of nature charac-terised by action, passion and drive.

Samana vayu: air or wind pervading the area between the navel and heart, and regulating digestion, assimilation of food, etc.

Sattva: one of the three gunas or essential qualities of nature characterised by purity, light and vital balance.

Shakti: the feminine, active, immanent, temporal principle.

Siddhis: psychic powers.

Sutras: lit. "thread"; aphorisms about the yogic life style compiled by the sage Patanjali.

Tamas: one of the three gunas or essential qualities of nature characterised by inaction, lethargy and darkness.

Trishula: Shiva's three-pointed weapon.

Udana vayu: air or wind pervading the head area, and regulating functions such as the blinking of the eyes, coughing, hiccups, and sneezing.

Ujjayi: "Victorious" breathing method practised by gently closing the glottis.

Vajra: ritual object in the Buddhist tradition.

Vayu: air or wind within the body; there are five of them and they need to flow unrestrictedly through our subtle energy paths in order to avoid disease.

Vedas: Hindu sacred scriptures from where all yoga originates.

Vijnanamaya kosha: lit. "wisdom sheath"; it corresponds to the intellect.

Vyana vayu: air or wind circulating throughout the body in all directions.

Yama: five ethical practices when relating to the outside world; first stage in Patanjali's eight-limbed path of yoga.

Yoga: lit. "to yoke or unite"; spiritual practice concerned with union.

Yogi/yogini: a person who practises yoga.

JOURNAL

Asana Index

JOURNAL

JOURNAL

JOURNAL

JOURNAL

JOURNAL

JOURNAL

JOURNAL

JOURNAL

JOURNAL

Lightning Source UK Ltd.
Milton Keynes UK
UKOW06f0454180214

226654UK00011B/32/P